MAXIMUM MASS

Eating to Dominate Your Opponent

Tim McClellan
Liz Sambach

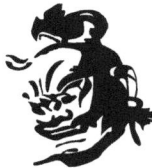

Budo Inc.

Library of Congress Cataloging - in - Publications Data.
McClellan, Tim
Maximum Mass: Eating to Dominate Your Opponent

Budo Incorporated
2815 E. Libra Street
Gilbert, AZ 85234

www.StrengthAndPeace.com

ACKNOWLEDGMENTS

KRISTLE SCHULZ
EDITOR/FORMATTING/GRAPHIC DESIGN

Without Kristle Schulz this project could not possibly have come to completion. Kristle did an outstanding job on Tim's previous books, *Inner Strength Inner Peace* and *Inner Strength Inner Peace II* so she was retained yet again to edit and provide all graphic design needs. With Kristle we always know things will be of the highest quality. Our appreciation and love for her is immense.

JUDD BIASIOTTO
NUTRITIONAL CONSULTANT

Dr. Judd is one of the most amazing men in history and his help with nutritional concepts can be described only as a blessing to us. Thank you Dr. Judd.

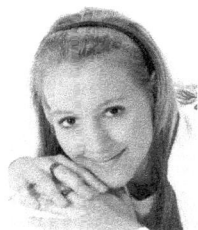

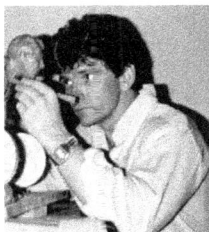

TABLE OF CONTENTS

CHAPTER 1

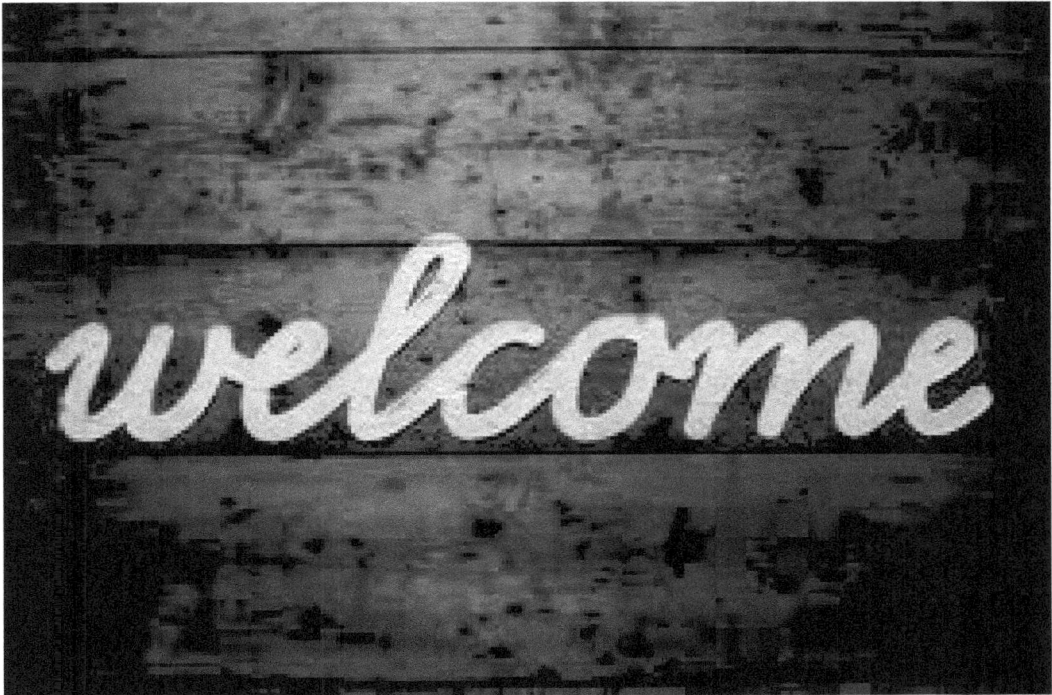

INTRODUCTION

You have selected us for weight gain advice. Thank you for your trust. You either are intellectually curious and seeking more wisdom, or you just want to get HUGE...perhaps SUPER HUGE. Cool. We're in. We can help you get huge, even super huge if you choose. We have done it before with others. We have even done it before with ourselves. We promise you, with diligent work, you can achieve these goals (this has to come from you, we cannot do this for you). It's going to take a little hard work, discipline and sacrifice, but you're old enough to now know anything worth having requires those efforts. Keep focused on the most important thing: the "after" picture of YOU. It's important to see daily, or several times daily, the outcome of your venture. Albert Einstein said, "Imagination is everything. It is a preview of life's coming attractions." He couldn't be more correct about that, which is why he gets the title of "super genius", and we don't. We do get other titles though, one of which is "successful at drastically changing bodies." Yes, we have coached athletes that have made mind-boggling changes with their physiques and we have done it in relatively short periods of time. By now, you can probably see we are quite confident in being able to help you change your body significantly because we have done it so many times before, over the course of decades.

DOES THIS DIET PLAN WORK?

Often ☑
Sometimes ☐
Seldom ☐
Never ☐

Yes, if you do. If you're compliant you should find yourself full of energy, very happy, huge and quite pleased with the results. Conversely, if you're one of those types that sits down to lunch on a diet of Big Macs or just tofu and other chic meal plans, then you might not see the same results as those who were better suited towards following vital directions (hereafter known as the ones that got the results they wanted). In short: you follow, you win. You cheat and you get the results cheaters deserve: small biceps and low power outputs. The results are up to only one person on earth, the same one who is responsible for what goes in your mouth: YOU. Choose wisely, like your body depends on it. We have and we're full of energy and happiness.

PROOF OF THIS PLAN'S EFFECTIVENESS

We are going to share a few stories about those who have made amazing changes in their body due to this meal plan. We won't tell too many as we don't want to waste a lot of your time. We're pretty much down-to-business types so we have tried to eliminate as much text as possible and have even condensed the bulk of the book into bullet points.

The first story starts in January of 2001. It involves a six-foot, seven-inches, 278-pound defensive end from the University of Illinois named Fred Wakefield. Fred was preparing for the annual N.F.L. Scouting Combine. He was obviously in a position to give his very best as he desperately wanted to get drafted and have a career in the N.F.L. Part of that process included a need to gain weight. In seven weeks, he gained twelve pounds, put forty pounds on his bench press and took three-tenths of a second off his 40-yard dash time. He even had a weightlifting photo published in USA Today. Look it up: it was the February 22, 2001 edition. That year he signed a contract with the Arizona Cardinals and found himself as a starter at defensive end that first season. The following year they wanted him to move inside to defense tackle, which would require additional weight gain. Again, he was able to gain that mass...well, that mass plus some. By the

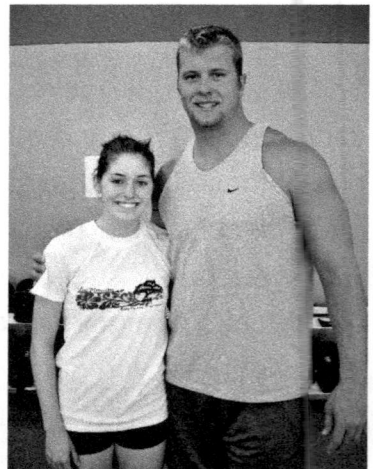

time Fred's career ended he was a rock-hard, lean, man-beast who weighed 330 pounds. The key there is that he was still lean. His work ethic and story was so inspirational Tim wrote a section on him in his second book, *Inner Strength Inner Peace II* (available at www.StrengthAndPeace.com).

Fast forward to 2007, same N.F.L. Combine training, only this time it's a beast of a tight end from Arizona State University named Zach Miller. Yes, this is *the* Zach Miller, the All-Pro tight end. Zach came in to his Combine prep an outstanding tight end, the best all-around tight end in the country. He just did not test out well, however, and the concern there is that it could drop his draft status and cost him millions of dollars. Zach chose a different route. He chose to think huge, eat huge, be huge. He gained thirteen pounds in seven weeks and doubled the number of reps he could do at 225 pounds in the bench press. He also added four inches to his vertical and ran his 40-yard dash three-tenths of a second faster. His story too is highlighted in *Inner Strength Inner Peace II* (still available at www.StrengthAndPeace.com in case you missed the first hint above).

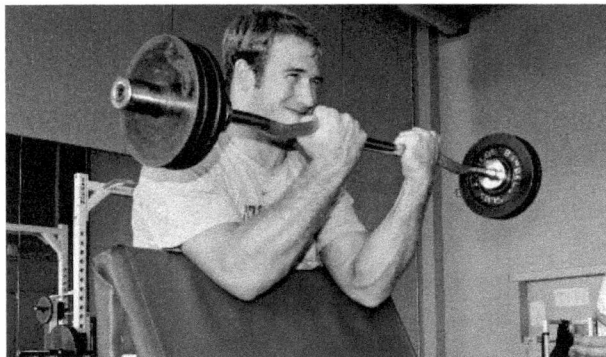

Time to get out of football and into something a little more serious: MMA. In this case we're talking about Mike VanArsdale, the cover boy for this book. Not a bad looking physique for a guy weighing in at 230 pounds, is it? What you may not realize is, at that same height (6'2") Mike won an NCAA national wrestling championship at 167 pounds! That's sixty-three pounds lighter, sixty-three less pounds of dominating mass. Who wouldn't love to gain muscle mass of that quality? It did not come easy for Mike. He lifted like a mad man and ate like a man who wanted to someday win a World Cup Championship in Freestyle wrestling. It took a lot of effort and dedication... but it was worth it.

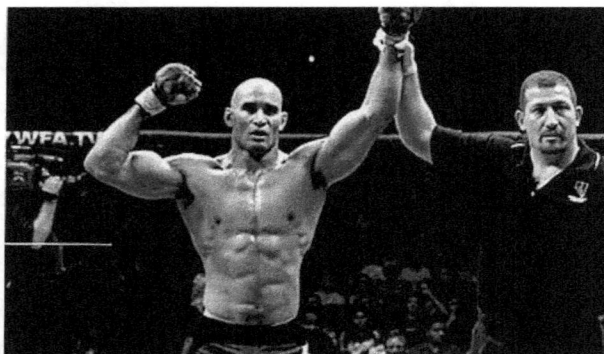

You just read two huge football success stories. Time for one more, this time a regular Joe...or a regular Tim. Tim was a second string, 148-pound junior wide receiver in high school. It was suggested to him by an outstanding coach of his, Tom Filipovits, that he gain weight (read a great story about him in *Inner Strength Inner Peace*. You can probably guess where you can find this book for sale). The following year Tim was a 200-pound All East Pennsylvania First Team honors recipient who was being recruited by colleges. A year later he was 230 pounds, playing college football and powerlifting.

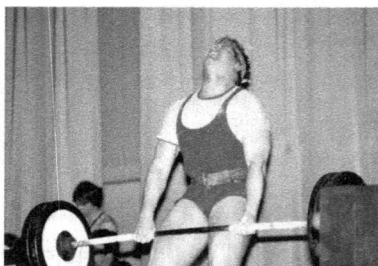
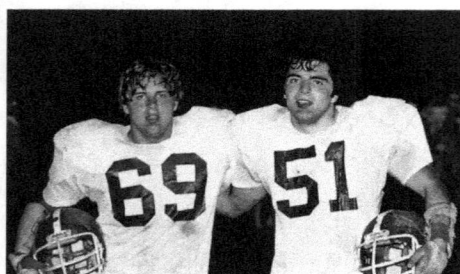

And finally, no, we are not sexist. One of us is, in fact, a female. We care about anyone who wants to gain some solid mass for performance domination, so here's one more success story. Liz was a natural athlete who played some softball, volleyball, basketball and track with normal success. She met a crew coach that told her if she gained weight she would be much better at crew. She did—the wrong way, hence becoming a self-described, 145-pound "fatty" (see below). With proper eating, she not only lost that "fatty" moniker but also gained fifteen pounds, earned a college scholarship to Gonzaga University and made All-Conference honors in crew. Talk about an amazing transition: from 145 pounds and kind of soft to 160 pounds of confident, hard-training, focused rowing stand-out.

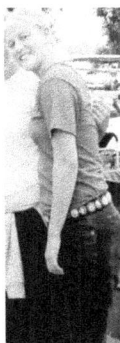

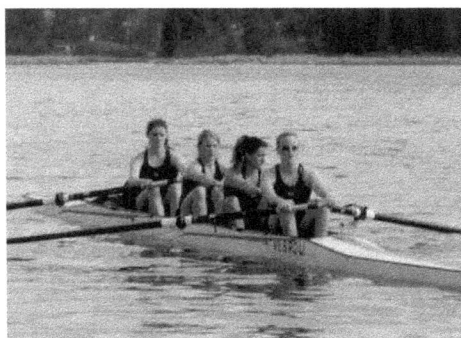

And just to let you know where it all ended: here's Liz, back down at 145 pounds, but no longer a self-described "fatty." You can now refer to her as r pped, or super fit.

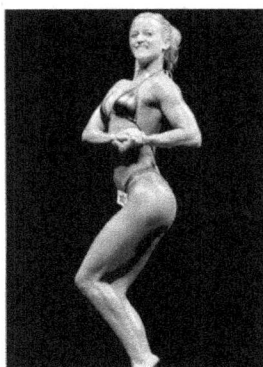

MORAL OF THE STORY

We've told you stories of NFL greats, MMA greats, high school athletes, gargantuan males, fatty females, ripped females and All-Pro players. Have you figured out what they all have in common? They followed the plan and they got huge results—the kind you want.

Need we say more? Remember who your outcome is up to and visualize that successful ending. It is a preview of a coming attraction, and that attraction will be you. Lets get to work. Think big, see big, be big. Sermon over. Amen.

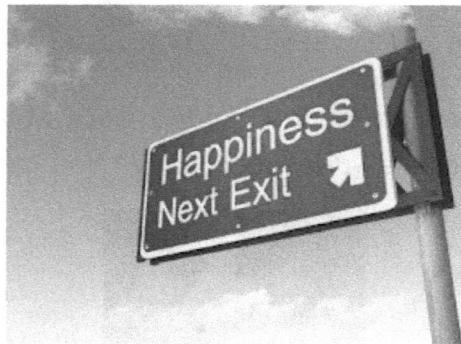

CHAPTER 2:

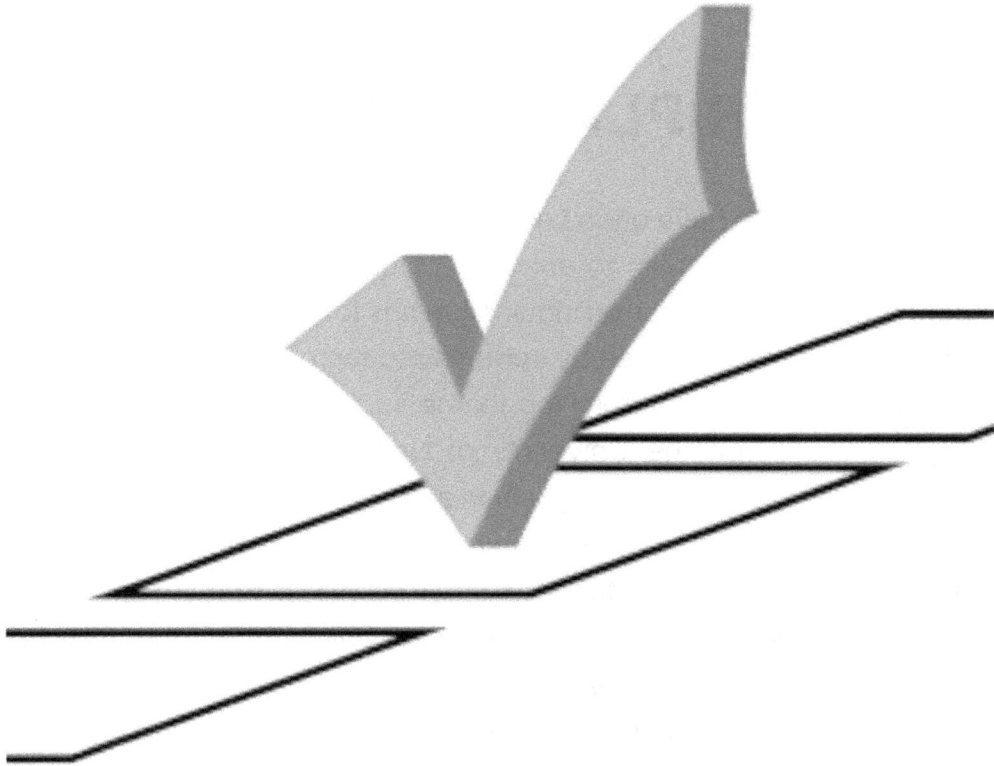

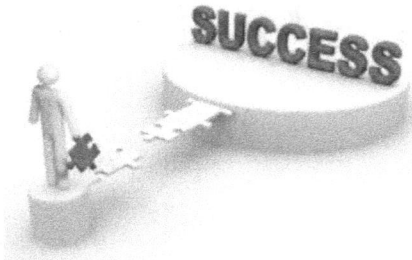

YOUR PLAN FOR SUCCESS

Over the years we have often been asked the question, "what should I eat?" We have tried everything to answer this question. To get this baseline of knowledge, we have referred inquiring minds to great best-selling books and provided documents written by some of the top performance enhancement specialists in the world, from top teams such as the Green Bay Packers, Stanford University, the University of Notre Dame and the New Jersey Devils, to name a few. The list goes on and on. We have also written detailed guidelines and constructed dynamic PowerPoint presentations. We hope each plan leads our athletes and other clients to greater understanding, self-empowerment and success. While we hate to admit our own failures, we have not been as successful as we would have liked to be through this approach. Why? Many of those who inquired don't necessarily want the knowledge for self-empowerment. They wanted to know *what to eat.*

For those of you who want to know what to eat: we have a treat for you—it's better than a Rice Krispie. This chapter is presenting a 21-day meal plan. It's all spelled out. It's child-proof. It's healthy. It is proven (refer back to the stories in the previous chapters if you skipped them—there is no skipping permitted in this plan). It will help you to make fabulous gains...if you follow it.

Since we promised to be respectful of your time and to minimize text, the meal plan follows. For those of you who are ready to start: "the pool's open, dive in." For those of you who seek better understanding of what you ingest, the chapters following the meal plan will give you the latest and greatest information on how to construct a healthy eating lifestyle that you can use forever. Not a bad trade-off for the price of the book…

Before we go any further, however, it's time for our C.Y.B. Notice:

In an extremely litigious society, it is important to continually cover your butt (C.Y.B.). Don't believe us? Consider this: In 1992, 79-year-old Stella Liebeck bought a cup of coffee at a McDonald's drive-thru in New Mexico and spilled it on her lap. She sued McDonald's. A jury awarded her nearly $3 million in punitive damages for the burns she suffered. Ouch, on both ends.

Therefore, we are not officially saying you should eat any of the foods on this meal plan. For all we know, you may have celiac disease and ingestion of wheat bread could cause you severe troubles. All we can say is: check with a doctor before eating any foods, breathing air, using medications you see on television commercials, etc. You can use this book for informative purposes with the understanding that, if it ends up on your lap, we will not be paying you 3 million dollars. We just don't have it. Seriously, now that our butts are covered, please do not eat any foods you may be allergic to, suspect you may have gastrointestinal problems with, etc. Thank you.

Bon appetite!

DAY ONE

Meal	Food	Amount	CAL	PRO	FAT	CHO	FIBER
1	Eggs	2 regular	155	13	11	1	0
	Whole Milk	1 cup	156	8	8	13	0
	Wheat Bread	2 slices	154	6	2	28	2
	Butter	1 TBSP	108	0	12	0	0
	Orange	1 medium	64	1	0	15	3
	Meal Totals		**637**	**28**	**33**	**57**	**5**
2	Grilled Chicken	4 ounces	113	26	1	0	0
	Wheat Bread	2 slices	154	6	2	28	2
	Low-fat Cheese	2 slices	92	14	4	0	0
	Meal Totals		**359**	**46**	**7**	**28**	**2**
3	Pineapple	1 cup	92	1	0	22	2
	Sandwiches:						
	Roast Beef	5 ounces	237	39	9	0	0
	Low-fat Cheese	2 slices	92	14	4	0	0
	Wheat Bread	4 slices	308	12	4	56	4
	Lettuce	1 cup	8	1	0	1	0
	Red Pepper	1/2 cup	24	1	0	5	1
	Meal Totals		**761**	**68**	**17**	**84**	**7**
4	Organic Peanut Butter	2 TBSP	200	8	16	6	3
	Red Apple	1 medium	76	0	0	19	3
	Muscle Milk	2 scoops	338	32	18	12	0
	Raspberries	1 cup	69	0	1	15	8
	Meal Totals		**683**	**40**	**35**	**52**	**14**

5	Ground Bison Burger	5 ounces	280	43	12	0	0
	Ketchup	4 TBSP	64	0	0	16	0
	Wheat Bun	1 bun (3.6 oz)	207	7	3	38	3
	Spinach	1 cup	8	1	0	1	1
	Brown Rice	1 cup	218	5	2	45	3
	Grape Juice	2 cups	336	0	0	84	0
	Meal Totals		**1113**	**56**	**17**	**184**	**7**
6	Greek Yogurt	1 container	108	15	0	12	0
	Honey	2 TBSP	140	0	0	35	0
	Pretzels	2 servings (2 oz)	200	4	0	46	2
	Meal Totals		**448**	**19**	**0**	**93**	**2**
	Daily Totals		**4001**	**257**	**109**	**498**	**37**

DAY TWO

Meal	Food	Amount	CAL	PRO	FAT	CHO	FIBER
1	Oatmeal	2 cups	276	12	4	48	8
	Whole Milk	2 cups	312	16	16	26	0
	Strawberries	1 cup	48	1	0	11	3
	Whey Protein Powder	1 scoop	104	20	0	6	0
	Meal Totals		**740**	**49**	**20**	**91**	**11**
2	Greek Yogurt	2 containers (10.6 oz)	216	30	0	24	0
	Almonds	1/4 cup	222	8	18	7	4
	Blueberry Juice	2 cups	224	0	0	56	0
	Meal Totals		**662**	**38**	**18**	**87**	**4**
3	Pineapple	1 cup	80	0	0	20	2
	Orange Juice	2 cups	224	4	0	52	0
	Sandwich:						
	Tuna	4 ounces	125	29	1	0	0
	Low-fat Cheese	2 slices	96	14	4	1	0
	Pumpernickel Bagel	1 (3.8 oz)	290	10	2	58	2
	Tomato	1 cup	40	2	0	8	2
	Lettuce	1 cup	8	1	0	1	0
	Meal Totals		**863**	**60**	**7**	**140**	**6**
4	Wheat Bread	2 slices	154	6	2	28	2
	Organic Almond Butter	2 TBSP	202	4	18	6	2
	Honey	1 TBSP	68	0	0	17	0
	Muscle Milk	2 scoops	338	32	18	12	0
	Meal Totals		**762**	**42**	**38**	**63**	**4**
5	Steak (T-bone)	5 ounces	238	37	10	0	0
	A-1 Steak Sauce	5 TBSP	60	0	0	16	0
	Green Beans	1 cup	36	2	0	7	3
	Sweet Potato	1 medium	100	2	0	23	2
	Meal Totals		**434**	**41**	**10**	**46**	**5**

6	Red Apple	1 medium	76	0	0	19	3
	Muscle Milk	1 scoop	169	16	9	6	0
	Graham Cracker	5 sheets	299	5	7	54	2
	Meal Totals		**544**	**21**	**16**	**79**	**5**
	Daily Totals		**4005**	**251**	**109**	**506**	**35**

DAY THREE

Meal	Food	Amount	CAL	PRO	FAT	CHO	FIBER
1	Rye Bread	2 slices	162	6	2	30	4
	Peanut Butter	2 TBSP	200	8	16	6	2
	Whey Protein Powder	2 scoops	208	40	0	12	0
	Orange Juice	2 cups	224	4	0	52	0
	Meal Totals		**794**	**58**	**18**	**100**	**6**
2	Muscle Milk	2 scoops	338	32	18	12	0
	Whole Wheat English Muffin	1 whole	141	6	1	27	4
	Peanut Butter	1 TBSP	100	4	8	3	1
	Honey	3 TBSP	208	0	0	52	0
	Meal Totals		**787**	**42**	**27**	**94**	**5**
3	Chicken	4 ounces	113	26	1	0	0
	Teriyaki Sauce	4 TBSP	64	4	0	12	0
	Quinoa	1 cup	224	8	4	39	5
	Broccoli (steamed)	1 cup	36	3	0	6	2
	Banana	1 regular	112	1	0	27	3
	Meal Totals		**549**	**42**	**5**	**84**	**10**
4	Greek Yogurt	2 containers (10.6oz)	216	30	0	24	0
	Almonds	1/4 cup	222	8	18	7	4
	Meal Totals		**438**	**38**	**18**	**31**	**4**
5	Ground Beef (95% lean)	6 ounces	217	34	9	0	0
	Wheat Pasta	1 cup, dry (3.7 oz)	385	15	1	79	9
	Marinara Sauce	1/2 cup	66	2	2	10	2
	Orange Juice	2 cups	224	4	0	52	0
	Meal Totals		**892**	**55**	**12**	**141**	**11**
6	Muscle Milk	2 scoops	338	32	18	12	0
	Pretzels	2 servings (2 oz)	200	4	0	46	2
	Meal Totals		**538**	**36**	**18**	**58**	**2**
	Daily Totals		**3998**	**271**	**98**	**508**	**38**

DAY FOUR

Meal	Food	Amount	CAL	PRO	FAT	CHO	FIBER
1	Eggs	2 regular	155	13	11	1	0
	Whole Milk	2 cups	312	16	16	26	0
	Cream of Wheat	2 cups	257	7	1	55	3
	Peach	1 medium	40	1	0	9	2
	Meal Totals		**764**	**37**	**28**	**91**	**5**
2	Greek Yogurt	2 containers (10.6 oz)	216	30	0	24	0
	Strawberry Preserves	4 TBSP	220	0	0	55	0
	Meal Totals		**436**	**30**	**0**	**79**	**0**
3	Mango	2 cups	225	3	1	51	5
	Sandwich:						
	Roast Beef	4 ounces	133	22	5	0	0
	Low-fat Cheese	2 slices	96	14	4	1	0
	Wheat Bread	2 slices	154	6	2	28	2
	Lettuce	1 cup	8	1	0	1	0
	Pepper	1/2 cup	24	1	0	5	1
	Meal Totals		**640**	**47**	**12**	**86**	**8**
4	Whole Milk	2 cups	312	16	16	26	0
	Peanuts	1/2 cup	363	36	19	12	6
	Banana	1 regular	112	1	0	27	3
	Meal Totals		**787**	**53**	**35**	**65**	**9**
5	Turkey Burger	6 ounces	254	32	14	0	0
	Ketchup	4 TBSP	64	0	0	16	0
	Wheat Bun	2 buns (5.2 ounces)	414	14	6	76	6
	Dill Pickle	3 slices (0.6 oz)	4	0	0	1	0
	Lettuce	1 cup	8	1	0	1	0
	Wild Rice	1 cup	173	6	1	35	3
	Meal Totals		**917**	**53**	**21**	**129**	**9**
6	Muscle Milk	1 scoop	169	16	9	6	0
	Strawberries	1 cup	48	1	0	11	3
	Blueberry Juice	2 cups	224	0	0	56	0
	Meal Totals		**441**	**17**	**9**	**73**	**3**
	Daily Totals		**3985**	**237**	**105**	**523**	**34**

DAY FIVE

Meal	Food	Amount	CAL	PRO	FAT	CHO	FIBER
1	Whole Wheat Waffles	4 waffles	356	10	12	52	6
	Honey	2 TBSP	140	0	0	35	0
	Organic Almond Butter	2 TBSP	202	4	18	6	2
	Muscle Milk	1 scoop	169	16	9	6	0
	Meal Totals		**867**	**30**	**39**	**99**	**8**
2	Greek Yogurt	2 containers (10.6 oz)	216	30	0	24	0
	Honey	1 TBSP	70	0	0	17	0
	Meal Totals		**286**	**30**	**0**	**41**	**0**
3	Chicken	6 ounces	169	39	2	0	0
	Baked Potato	1 medium	164	4	0	37	4
	Cheddar Cheese	1/4 cup (shredded)	109	7	9	0	0
	Banana	1 regular	112	1	0	27	3
	Low-fat Chocolate Milk	1 cup	154	8	2	26	1
	Meal Totals		**708**	**59**	**13**	**90**	**8**
4	Graham Cracker	5 sheets	299	5	7	54	2
	Whey Protein Powder	2 scoops	208	40	0	12	0
	Organic Peanut Butter	2 TBSP	200	8	16	6	2
	Meal Totals		**707**	**53**	**23**	**72**	**4**
5	Lean Beef Steak	6 ounces	232	40	8	0	0
	Brown Rice	2 cups	428	10	4	88	6
	Cauliflower	1 cup	32	2	0	6	3
	Green Beans	1 cup	36	2	0	7	3
	Grape Juice	1 cup	168	0	0	42	0
	Meal Totals		**896**	**54**	**12**	**143**	**12**
6	Muscle Milk	2 scoops	338	32	18	12	0
	Blueberries	2 cups	189	2	1	43	7
	Meal Totals		**527**	**34**	**19**	**55**	**7**
	Daily Totals		**3991**	**260**	**106**	**500**	**39**

DAY SIX

Meal	Food	Amount	CAL	PRO	FAT	CHO	FIBER
1	Whey Protein Powder	2 scoops	208	40	0	12	0
	Cream of Wheat	2 cups	257	7	1	55	3
	Whole Milk	2 cups	312	16	16	26	0
	Raspberries	1 cup	69	0	1	15	8
	Meal Totals		**846**	**63**	**18**	**108**	**11**
2	Low-fat String Cheese	2 sticks	154	16	10	0	0
	Muscle Milk	2 scoops	338	32	18	12	0
	Green Apple	1 medium	76	0	0	19	3
	Meal Totals		**568**	**48**	**28**	**31**	**3**
3	Ground Bison Burger	6 ounces	334	52	14	0	0
	Spinach	2 cups	16	2	0	2	2
	Mushrooms	1 cup	16	2	0	2	1
	Quinoa	1/2 cup	110	4	2	19	2
	Blueberry Juice	1 cup	112	0	0	28	0
	Meal Totals		**588**	**60**	**16**	**51**	**5**
4	Greek Yogurt	2 containers	216	30	0	24	0
	Honey	2 TBSP	140	0	0	35	0
	Strawberry Preserves	4 TBSP	220	0	0	55	0
	Meal Totals		**576**	**30**	**0**	**114**	**0**
5	Ham (Extra Lean Steak)	4 ounces	185	25	9	1	0
	Baked Beans	1/2 cup	146	7	2	25	7
	Sweet Potato	1 medium	100	2	0	23	2
	Butter	1 TBSP	108	0	12	0	0
	Orange Juice	2 cups	224	4	0	52	0
	Meal Totals		**763**	**38**	**23**	**101**	**9**
6	Mango	2 cups	225	3	1	51	5
	Muscle Milk	2 scoops	338	32	18	12	0
	Blueberries	1 cup	88	1	0	21	4
	Meal Totals		**651**	**36**	**19**	**84**	**9**
	Daily Totals		**3992**	**275**	**104**	**489**	**37**

DAY SEVEN

Meal	Food	Amount	CAL	PRO	FAT	CHO	FIBER
1	Whole Wheat English Muffin	2 muffins (2.3 oz)	287	12	3	53	9
	Eggs	4 regular	293	25	21	1	0
	Orange Juice	2 cups	224	4	0	52	0
	Plums	2 medium	64	0	0	16	2
	Meal Totals		**868**	**41**	**24**	**122**	**11**
2	Greek Yogurt	2 containers	216	30	0	24	0
	Whey Protein Powder	2 scoops	208	40	0	12	0
	Meal Totals		**424**	**70**	**0**	**36**	**0**
3	Chicken	4 ounces	113	26	1	0	0
	Teriyaki Sauce	4 TBSP	64	4	0	12	0
	Wild Rice	2 cups	346	12	2	70	6
	Broccoli (steamed)	1 cup	24	2	0	4	2
	Carrots	1 cup	56	2	0	12	4
	Apple Juice	2 cups	232	0	0	58	0
	Meal Totals		**835**	**46**	**3**	**156**	**12**
4	Rye Bread	2 slices	162	6	2	30	4
	Organic Peanut Butter	2 TBSP	200	8	16	6	2
	Honey	2 TBSP	140	0	0	35	0
	Meal Totals		**502**	**14**	**18**	**71**	**6**
5	Salmon	4 ounces	200	23	12	0	0
	Spinach	1 cup	8	1	0	1	1
	Cauliflower	1 cup	32	2	0	6	3
	Baked Potato	1 medium	164	4	0	37	4
	Whole Milk	2 cups	312	16	16	26	0
	Meal Totals		**716**	**46**	**28**	**70**	**8**
6	Muscle Milk	2 scoops	338	32	18	12	0
	Pretzels	2 servings (2 oz)	200	4	0	46	2
	Meal Totals		**538**	**36**	**18**	**58**	**2**
	Daily Totals		**3883**	**253**	**91**	**513**	**39**

DAY EIGHT

Meal	Food	Amount	CAL	PRO	FAT	CHO	FIBER
1	Eggs	4 large	275	25	19	1	0
	Spinach	1 cup	8	1	0	1	1
	Tomato	1/2 cup	20	1	0	4	1
	Peppers	1/2 cup	24	1	0	5	1
	Low-fat Cheese	2 slices	92	14	4	0	0
	Whole Wheat Pita	2 large	355	12	3	70	9
	Meal Totals		**774**	**54**	**26**	**81**	**12**
2	Muscle Milk	2 scoops	338	32	18	12	0
	Graham Crackers	5 sheets	299	5	7	54	2
	Meal Totals		**637**	**37**	**25**	**66**	**2**
3	Sandwiches:						
	Ground Bison Burger	6 ounces	325	52	13	0	0
	Ketchup	4 TBSP	64	0	0	16	0
	Low-fat Cheese	2 slices	92	14	4	0	0
	Wheat Bun	2 buns (5.2 ounces)	414	14	6	76	6
	Spinach	1/2 cup	8	1	0	1	1
	Tomato	1/2 cup	20	1	0	4	1
	Meal Totals		**923**	**82**	**23**	**97**	**8**
4	Greek Yogurt	2 containers	216	30	0	24	0
	Pretzels	2 servings (2 oz)	200	4	0	46	2
	Meal Totals		**416**	**34**	**0**	**70**	**2**
5	Lean Beef Steak	4 ounces	153	27	5	0	0
	A-1 Steak Sauce	6 TBSP	72	0	0	18	0
	Spaghetti Squash	2 cups	88	2	0	20	4
	Wild Rice	2 cups	346	12	2	70	6
	Grape Juice	1 1/2 cups	252	0	0	63	0
	Meal Totals		**911**	**41**	**7**	**171**	**10**
6	Red Apple	1 medium	76	0	0	19	3
	Low-fat String Cheese	2 sticks	154	16	10	0	0
	Muscle Milk	1 scoop	169	16	9	6	0
	Meal Totals		**399**	**32**	**19**	**25**	**3**
	Daily Totals		**4060**	**280**	**100**	**510**	**37**

DAY NINE

Meal	Food	Amount	CAL	PRO	FAT	CHO	FIBER
1	Oatmeal	2 cups	284	12	4	50	8
	Brown Sugar	4 TSP (packed)	72	0	0	18	0
	Muscle Milk	2 scoops	338	32	18	12	0
	Banana	1 regular	112	1	0	27	3
	Meal Totals		**806**	**45**	**22**	**107**	**11**
2	Whole Wheat English Muffin	1 muffin	141	6	1	27	4
	Turkey	4 ounces	110	19	2	4	0
	Whole Milk	2 cups	312	16	16	26	0
	Meal Totals		**563**	**41**	**19**	**57**	**4**
3	Grilled Chicken	4 ounces	113	26	1	0	0
	Wheat Bread	2 slices	141	6	1	27	2
	Spinach	1/2 cup	8	1	0	1	1
	Pretzels	3 servings (3 oz)	300	6	0	69	3
	Meal Totals		**562**	**39**	**2**	**97**	**6**
4	Greek Yogurt	1 container (5.3 oz)	108	15	0	12	0
	Honey	2 TBSP	140	0	0	35	0
	Blueberry Juice	2 cups	224	0	0	56	0
	Whey Protein Powder	2 scoops	208	40	0	12	0
	Meal Totals		**680**	**55**	**0**	**115**	**0**
5	Ham (Extra Lean Steak)	4 ounces	185	25	9	1	0
	Baked Potato	1 medium	164	4	0	37	4
	Baked Beans	1/2 cup	146	7	2	25	7
	Cheddar Cheese	1/4 cup (shredded)	109	7	9	0	0
	Sour Cream	1/4 cup	124	2	12	2	0
	Meal Totals		**728**	**45**	**32**	**65**	**11**
6	Graham Crackers	5 sheets	299	5	7	54	2
	Whey Protein Powder	2 scoops	208	40	0	12	0
	Organic Almond Butter	2 TBSP	202	4	18	6	2
	Meal Totals		**709**	**49**	**25**	**72**	**4**
	Daily Totals		**4048**	**274**	**100**	**513**	**36**

DAY TEN

Meal	Food	Amount	CAL	PRO	FAT	CHO	FIBER
1	Whole Wheat Waffles	2 waffles	178	5	6	26	3
	Organic Peanut Butter	2 TBSP	200	8	16	6	2
	Whole Milk	2 cups	312	16	16	26	0
	Meal Totals		**690**	**29**	**38**	**58**	**5**
2	Wheat Bread	2 slices	154	6	2	28	2
	Organic Almond Butter	1 TBSP	101	2	9	3	1
	Raisins	1/4 cup	136	1	0	33	1
	Honey	1 TBSP	68	0	0	17	0
	Whey Protein Powder	2 scoops	208	40	0	12	0
	Orange Juice	1 cup	112	2	0	26	0
	Meal Totals		**779**	**51**	**11**	**119**	**4**
3	Ground Beef (95% lean)	6 ounces	217	34	9	0	0
	Wheat Pasta	1 cup, dry (3.7 oz)	385	15	1	79	9
	Marinara Sauce	1 cup	66	2	2	10	3
	Grape Juice	1 cup	168	0	0	42	0
	Meal Totals		**836**	**51**	**12**	**131**	**12**
4	Muscle Milk	2 scoops	338	32	18	12	0
	Banana	1 regular	112	1	0	27	3
	Meal Totals		**450**	**33**	**18**	**39**	**3**
5	Roast Beef	6 ounces	195	33	7	0	0
	Ketchup	4 TBSP	64	0	0	16	0
	Wheat Bun	2 buns (5.2 ounces)	414	14	6	76	6
	Sweet Potato	1 medium	100	2	0	23	2
	Broccoli (steamed)	1 cup	24	2	0	4	2
	Meal Totals		**797**	**51**	**13**	**119**	**10**
6	Whey Protein Powder	2 scoops	208	40	0	12	0
	Graham Cracker	5 sheets	239	4	6	44	2
	Meal Totals		**447**	**44**	**6**	**56**	**2**
	Daily Totals		**3999**	**259**	**98**	**522**	**36**

DAY ELEVEN

Meal	Food	Amount	CAL	PRO	FAT	CHO	FIBER
1	Whole Milk	2 cups	312	16	16	26	0
	Cream of Wheat	1 cup	128	4	0	28	1
	Banana	1 regular	112	1	0	27	3
	Whey Protein Powder	1 scoop	104	20	0	6	0
	Raisins	1/2 cup (packed)	268	2	0	65	3
	Meal Totals		**924**	**43**	**16**	**152**	**7**
2	Low-fat Cottage Cheese	1 cup	154	28	2	6	0
	Strawberries	1 cup	48	1	0	11	3
	Muscle Milk	1 scoop	169	16	9	6	0
	Meal Totals		**371**	**45**	**11**	**23**	**3**
3	Sandwich:						
	Ham (Extra Lean Steak)	5 ounces	231	31	11	1	0
	Low-fat Cheese	1 slice	46	7	2	0	0
	Ketchup	4 TBSP	64	0	0	16	0
	Rye Bread	2 slices	162	6	2	30	4
	Lettuce	1 cup	8	1	0	1	0
	Apple Juice	2 cups	232	0	0	58	0
	Meal Totals		**743**	**45**	**15**	**106**	**4**
4	Whole Wheat Pita	2 large	355	12	3	70	9
	Ground Beef	6 ounces	217	34	9	0	0
	Lettuce	1 cup	8	1	0	1	0
	Yellow Mustard	to taste	0	0	0	0	0
	Meal Totals		**580**	**47**	**12**	**71**	**9**
5	Salmon	6 ounces	300	38	16	0	0
	Teriyaki Sauce	5 TBSP	80	5	0	15	0
	Green Beans	1 cup	36	2	0	7	3
	Butter	1 TBSP	108	0	12	0	0
	Baked Potato	1 medium	164	4	0	37	4
	Meal Totals		**688**	**49**	**28**	**59**	**7**

6	Pretzels	3 servings (3 oz)	300	6	0	69	3
	Plum	2 medium	64	0	0	16	2
	Muscle Milk	2 scoops	338	32	18	12	0
	Meal Totals		**702**	**38**	**18**	**97**	**5**
	Daily Totals		**4008**	**267**	**100**	**508**	**35**

DAY TWELVE

Meal	Food	Amount	CAL	PRO	FAT	CHO	FIBER
1	Whole Wheat English Muffin	2 muffins (2.3 oz)	287	12	3	53	9
	Butter	1 TBSP	108	0	12	0	0
	Muscle Milk	2 scoops	338	32	18	12	0
	Orange Juice	2 cups	224	4	0	52	0
	Meal Totals		**957**	**48**	**33**	**117**	**9**
2	Roast Beef	6 ounces	195	33	7	0	0
	Rye Bread	2 slices	162	6	2	32	4
	Lettuce	1 cup	8	1	0	1	0
	Yellow Mustard	to taste	0	0	0	0	0
	Meal Totals		**365**	**40**	**9**	**31**	**4**
3	Sandwiches:						
	Turkey Burger	6 ounces	254	32	14	1	0
	Ketchup	4 TBSP	64	0	0	16	0
	Wheat Bun	2 buns (5.2 ounces)	414	14	6	76	6
	Lettuce	1 cup	8	1	0	1	0
	Pepper	1/2 cup	24	1	0	5	1
	Brown Rice	1 cup	214	5	2	44	3
	Meal Totals		**978**	**53**	**22**	**142**	**10**
4	Pumpernickel Bagel	1 (3.8 oz)	290	10	2	58	2
	Whey Protein Powder	1 scoop	104	20	0	6	0
	Organic Peanut Butter	2 TBSP	200	8	16	6	2
	Meal Totals		**594**	**38**	**18**	**70**	**4**
5	Lean Beef Steak	8 ounces	311	53	11	0	0
	A-1 Steak Sauce	6 TBSP	72	0	0	18	0
	Cauliflower	1 cup	32	2	0	6	3
	Sweet Potato	1 med	100	2	0	23	2
	Meal Totals		**515**	**57**	**11**	**47**	**5**
6	Muscle Milk	1 scoop	169	16	9	6	0
	Graham Crackers	5 sheets	299	5	7	54	2
	Strawberry Preserves	2 TBSP	110	0	0	27	0
	Meal Totals		**578**	**21**	**16**	**87**	**2**
	Daily Totals		**3987**	**257**	**109**	**494**	**34**

DAY THIRTEEN

Mea	Food	Amount	CAL	PRO	FAT	CHO	FIBER
1	Oatmeal	1 cup	142	6	2	25	4
	Almonds	1/4 cup	222	8	18	7	4
	Whey Protein Powder	2 scoops	208	40	0	12	0
	Brown Sugar	4 TSP (packed)	72	0	0	18	0
	Orange Juice	2 cups	224	4	0	52	0
	Meal Totals		**868**	**58**	**20**	**114**	**8**
2	Greek Yogurt	2 containers (10.6 oz)	216	30	0	24	0
	Honey	2 TBSP	140	0	0	35	0
	Meal Totals		**356**	**30**	**0**	**59**	**0**
3	Sandwiches:						
	Ground Bison Burger	5 ounces	280	43	12	0	0
	Ketchup	4 TBSP	64	0	0	16	0
	Low-fat Cheese	2 slices	92	14	4	0	0
	Whole Wheat Pita	2 large	355	12	3	70	9
	Meal Totals		**791**	**69**	**19**	**86**	**9**
4	Muscle Milk	2 scoops	338	32	18	12	0
	Banana	1 regular	112	1	0	27	3
	Meal Totals		**450**	**33**	**18**	**39**	**3**
5	Turkey Burger	6 ounces	254	32	14	0	0
	Ketchup	4 TBSP	64	0	0	16	0
	Wheat Bun	2 buns (5.2 ounces)	414	14	6	76	6
	Wild Rice	2 cups	346	12	2	70	6
	Baked Beans	1/2 cup	138	6	2	24	6
	Meal Totals		**1216**	**64**	**24**	**186**	**18**
6	Muscle Milk	2 scoops	338	32	18	12	0
	Meal Totals		**338**	**32**	**18**	**12**	**0**
	Daily Totals		**4019**	**286**	**99**	**496**	**38**

DAY FOURTEEN

Meal	Food	Amount	CAL	PRO	FAT	CHO	FIBER
1	Whole Wheat Waffles	2 waffles	178	5	6	26	3
	Strawberries	1 cup	48	1	0	11	3
	Organic Almond Butter	2 TBSP	210	4	18	8	2
	Muscle Milk	2 scoops	320	32	16	12	0
	Meal Totals		**756**	**42**	**40**	**57**	**8**
2	Greek Yogurt	2 containers (10.6 oz)	216	30	0	24	0
	Honey	4 TBSP	280	0	0	70	0
	Meal Totals		**496**	**30**	**0**	**94**	**0**
3	Sandwich:						
	Tuna	4 ounces	125	29	1	0	0
	Low-fat Cheese	2 slices	92	14	4	0	0
	Pumpernickel Bagel	1 (2.8)	290	10	2	58	2
	Tomato	1 cup	40	2	0	8	2
	Dill Pickle	3 slices (0.6 oz)	4	0	0	1	0
	Lettuce	1 cup	8	1	0	1	0
	Orange Juice	2 cups	224	4	0	52	0
	Meal Totals		**783**	**60**	**7**	**120**	**4**
4	Pretzels	3 servings (3 oz)	300	6	0	69	3
	Grilled Chicken	4 ounces	113	26	1	0	0
	Apple Juice	2 cups	232	0	0	58	0
	Meal Totals		**645**	**32**	**1**	**127**	**3**
5	Steak (T-bone)	6 ounces	288	45	12	0	0
	Teriyaki Sauce	5 TBSP	80	5	0	15	0
	Green Beans	1 cup	36	2	0	7	3
	Baked Potato	1 medium	164	4	0	37	4
	Meal Totals		**568**	**56**	**12**	**59**	**7**
6	Red Apple	1 medium	76	0	0	19	3
	Muscle Milk	2 scoops	338	32	18	12	0
	Whole Milk	2 cups	312	16	16	26	0
	Meal Totals		**726**	**48**	**34**	**57**	**3**
	Daily Totals		**3974**	**268**	**94**	**514**	**25**

DAY FIFTEEN

Meal	Food	Amount	CAL	PRO	FAT	CHO	FIBER
1	Eggs	4 large	275	25	19	1	0
	Brown Sugar	4 TSP (packed)	72	0	0	18	0
	Cream of Wheat	2 cups	257	7	1	55	3
	Strawberries	2 cups	96	2	0	22	6
	Meal Totals		**700**	**34**	**20**	**96**	**9**
2	Greek Yogurt	2 containers (10.6 oz)	216	30	0	24	0
	Mango	2 cups	225	3	1	51	5
	Meal Totals		**441**	**33**	**1**	**75**	**5**
3	Sandwich:						
	Roast Beef	4 ounces	133	22	5	0	0
	Low-fat Cheese	2 slices	96	14	4	1	0
	Rye Bread	2 slices	162	6	2	30	4
	Blueberry Juice	1 cup	112	0	0	28	0
	Meal Totals		**503**	**42**	**11**	**59**	**4**
4	Whey Protein Powder	2 scoops	208	40	0	12	0
	Almonds	1/4 cup	222	8	18	7	4
	Meal Totals		**430**	**48**	**18**	**19**	**4**
5	Hamburger	8 ounces	290	45	12	0	0
	Ketchup	4 TBSP	64	0	0	16	0
	Wheat Bun	2 buns (5.2 ounces)	414	14	6	76	6
	Lettuce	1 cup	8	1	0	1	0
	Dill Pickle	3 slices (0.6 oz)	4	0	0	1	0
	Quinoa	1 cup	224	8	4	39	5
	Grape Juice	2 cups	336	0	0	84	0
	Meal Totals		**1340**	**68**	**22**	**217**	**11**
6	Muscle Milk	2 scoops	338	32	18	12	0
	Low-fat String Cheese	2 sticks	154	16	10	0	0
	Peach	2 medium	80	2	0	18	4
	Meal Totals		**572**	**50**	**28**	**30**	**4**
	Daily Totals		**3986**	**275**	**100**	**496**	**37**

DAY SIXTEEN

Meal	Food	Amount	CAL	PRO	FAT	CHO	FIBER
1	Whey Protein Powder	2 scoops	208	40	0	12	0
	Oatmeal	1 cup	142	6	2	25	4
	Honey	2 TBSP	140	0	0	35	0
	Grape Juice	2 cups	336	0	0	84	0
	Meal Totals		**826**	**46**	**2**	**156**	**4**
2	Low-fat String Cheese	1 stick	77	8	5	0	0
	Muscle Milk	2 scoops	338	32	18	12	0
	Meal Totals		**415**	**40**	**23**	**12**	**0**
3	Ground Bison Burger	6 ounces	420	65	18	0	0
	Spinach	1 cup	16	2	0	2	2
	Brown Rice	1 cup	214	5	2	44	3
	Meal Totals		**650**	**72**	**20**	**46**	**5**
4	Greek Yogurt	2 containers	216	30	0	24	0
	Pretzels	2 servings (2 oz)	200	4	0	46	2
	Mango	2 cups	225	3	1	51	5
	Meal Totals		**641**	**37**	**1**	**121**	**7**
5	Ham (Extra Lean Steak)	6 ounces	231	25	11	1	0
	Cauliflower	1 cup	32	2	0	6	3
	Tomato	1 cup	40	2	0	8	2
	Sweet Potato	1 medium	100	2	0	23	2
	Butter	2 TBSP	207	0	23	0	0
	Grape Juice	2 cups	336	0	0	84	0
	Meal Totals		**946**	**31**	**34**	**122**	**7**
6	Raspberries	2 cups	138	0	2	30	16
	Muscle Milk	2 scoops	338	32	18	12	0
	Meal Totals		**476**	**32**	**20**	**42**	**16**
	Daily Totals		**3954**	**258**	**100**	**499**	**39**

DAY SEVENTEEN

Meal	Food	Amount	CAL	PRO	FAT	CHO	FIBER
1	Eggs	4 regular	310	26	22	2	0
	Apple Juice	2 cups	232	0	0	58	0
	Rye Toast	4 slices	324	12	4	60	8
	Meal Totals		**866**	**38**	**26**	**120**	**8**
2	Turkey	4 ounces	114	19	2	5	1
	Whole Wheat English Muffin	1 muffin (1.1 oz)	141	6	1	27	4
	Lettuce	1 cup	8	1	0	1	0
	Yellow Mustard	to taste	0	0	0	0	0
	Muscle Milk	2 scoops	338	32	18	12	0
	Meal Totals		**601**	**58**	**21**	**45**	**5**
3	Sandwich:						
	Grilled Chicken	6 ounces	174	39	2	0	0
	Wheat Bread	2 slices	154	6	2	28	2
	Lettuce	1 cup	8	1	0	1	0
	Red Pepper	1/2 cup	24	1	0	5	1
	Orange Juice	2 cups	224	4	0	52	0
	Meal Totals		**584**	**51**	**4**	**86**	**3**
4	Organic Peanut Butter	2 TBSP	200	8	16	6	2
	Graham Cracker	5 sheets	299	5	7	54	2
	Whey Protein Powder	2 scoops	208	40	0	12	0
	Meal Totals		**707**	**53**	**23**	**72**	**4**
5	Steak (T-bone)	6 ounces	288	45	12	0	0
	Spinach	1 cup	16	2	0	2	2
	Spaghetti Squash	1 cup	44	1	0	10	2
	Wild Rice	2 cups	346	12	2	70	6
	Blueberry Juice	2 cups	224	0	0	56	0
	Meal Totals		**918**	**60**	**14**	**138**	**10**
6	Muscle Milk	1 scoop	169	16	9	6	0
	Strawberries	2 cups	96	2	0	22	6
	Pretzels	1 serving (1 oz)	100	2	0	23	1
	Meal Totals		**365**	**20**	**9**	**51**	**7**
	Daily Totals		**4041**	**280**	**97**	**512**	**37**

DAY EIGHTEEN

Meal	Food	Amount	CAL	PRO	FAT	CHC	FIBER
1	Muscle Milk	1 scoop	169	16	9	6	0
	Skim Milk	1 cup	80	8	0	12	0
	Pumpernickel Bagel	1 (2.8 oz)	290	10	2	58	2
	Butter	1 TBSP	108	0	12	0	0
	Orange Juice	1 cup	112	2	0	26	0
	Meal Totals		**759**	**36**	**23**	**102**	**2**
2	Organic Almond Butter	2 TBSP	211	4	19	6	2
	Whole Wheat Pita	2 large	355	12	3	70	9
	Honey	4 TBSP	280	0	0	70	0
	Meal Totals		**846**	**16**	**22**	**146**	**11**
3	Ground Bison Burger	6 ounces	420	65	18	0	0
	Ketchup	4 TBSP	64	0	0	16	0
	Wheat Bread	2 slices	154	6	2	28	2
	Lettuce	1 cup	8	1	0	1	0
	Carrot	10 baby carrots	56	2	0	12	4
	Meal Totals		**702**	**74**	**20**	**57**	**6**
4	Whole Milk	2 cups	312	16	16	26	0
	Muscle Milk	1 scoop	169	16	9	6	0
	Meal Totals		**481**	**32**	**25**	**32**	**0**
5	Salmon	6 ounces	300	38	16	0	0
	Wheat Pasta	1 cup, dry (3.7 oz)	385	15	1	79	9
	Broccoli (steamed)	1 cup	24	2	0	4	2
	Apple Juice	1 cup	116	0	0	29	0
	Meal Totals		**825**	**55**	**17**	**112**	**11**
6	Greek Yogurt	1 container (5.3 oz)	84	15	0	6	0
	Blueberries	2 cups	189	2	1	43	7
	Whey Protein Powder	2 scoops	208	40	0	12	0
	Meal Totals		**481**	**57**	**1**	**61**	**7**
	Daily Totals		**4094**	**270**	**108**	**510**	**37**

DAY NINETEEN

Meal	Food	Amount	CAL	PRO	FAT	CHO	FIBER
1	Oatmeal	2 cups	284	12	4	50	8
	Greek Yogurt	2 containers (10.6 oz)	216	30	0	24	0
	Brown Sugar	4 TSP (packed)	72	0	0	18	0
	Whole Milk	2 cups	312	16	16	26	0
	Meal Totals		**884**	**58**	**20**	**118**	**8**
2	Wheat Bread	2 slices	154	6	2	28	2
	Organic Peanut Butter	2 TBSP	200	8	16	6	2
	Honey	2 TBSP	140	0	0	35	0
	Whey Protein Powder	2 scoops	208	40	0	12	0
	Meal Totals		**702**	**54**	**18**	**81**	**4**
3	Grilled Chicken	4 ounces	113	26	1	0	0
	Ketchup	4 TBSP	64	0	0	16	0
	Low-Fat Cheese	2 slices	92	14	4	0	0
	Wheat Bread	2 slices	154	6	2	28	2
	Lettuce	1 cup	8	1	0	1	0
	Pretzels	3 servings (3 oz)	300	6	0	69	3
	Meal Totals		**731**	**53**	**7**	**114**	**5**
4	Muscle Milk	2 scoops	338	32	18	12	0
	Banana	1 regular	112	1	0	27	3
	Orange Juice	1 cup	112	2	0	26	0
	Meal Totals		**562**	**35**	**18**	**65**	**3**
5	Shrimp	6 ounces	181	34	5	0	0
	Spinach	1 cup	16	2	0	2	2
	Carrots	1 cup	56	2	0	12	4
	Spaghetti Squash	1 cup	44	1	0	10	2
	Brown Rice	2 cups	428	10	4	88	6
	Butter	1 TBSP	108	0	12	0	0
	Meal Totals		**833**	**49**	**21**	**112**	**14**
6	Muscle Milk	2 scoops	338	32	18	12	0
	Meal Totals		**338**	**32**	**18**	**12**	**0**
	Daily Totals		**4050**	**281**	**102**	**502**	**34**

DAY TWENTY

Meal	Food	Amount	CAL	PRO	FAT	CHO	FIBER
1	Whole Wheat Waffles	2 waffles	178	5	6	26	3
	Organic Almond Butter	2 TBSP	202	4	18	6	2
	Whey Protein Powder	2 scoops	208	40	0	12	0
	Honey	2 TBSP	140	0	0	35	0
	Meal Totals		**728**	**49**	**24**	**79**	**5**
2	Greek Yogurt	2 containers (10.6oz)	216	30	0	24	0
	Mango	1 cup	104	1	0	25	2
	Meal Totals		**320**	**31**	**0**	**49**	**2**
3	Roast Beef	6 ounces	249	42	9	0	0
	Rye Bread	2 slices	162	6	2	30	4
	Tomato	1/2 cup	20	1	0	4	1
	Lettuce	1 cup	8	1	0	1	0
	Grape Juice	2 cups	336	0	0	84	0
	Meal Totals		**775**	**50**	**11**	**119**	**5**
4	Muscle Milk	2 scoops	338	32	18	12	0
	Orange	1 medium	76	1	0	18	3
	Meal Totals		**414**	**33**	**18**	**30**	**3**
5	Turkey Burger	6 ounces	254	32	14	0	0
	Ketchup	4 TBSP	64	0	0	16	0
	Wheat Bun	2 buns (5.2 ounces)	414	14	6	76	6
	Wild Rice	2 cups	346	12	2	70	6
	Baked Beans	1/2 cup	138	6	2	24	6
	Meal Totals		**1216**	**64**	**24**	**186**	**18**
6	Banana	1 regular	112	1	0	27	3
	Muscle Milk	2 scoops	338	32	18	12	0
	Meal Totals		**450**	**33**	**18**	**39**	**3**
	Daily Totals		**3903**	**260**	**95**	**502**	**36**

DAY TWENTY-ONE

Mea	Food	Amount	CAL	PRO	FAT	CHO	FIBER
1	Eggs	4 large	275	25	19	1	0
	Spinach	1 cup	16	2	0	2	2
	Low-fat Cheese	2 slices	96	14	4	1	0
	Whole Wheat English Muffin	2 muffins (2.3 oz)	287	12	3	53	9
	Orange Juice	2 cups	224	4	0	52	0
	Meal Totals		**898**	**57**	**26**	**109**	**11**
2	Grilled Chicken	6 ounces	174	39	2	0	0
	Wheat Bread	2 slices	154	6	2	28	2
	Grape Juice	2 cups	336	0	0	84	0
	Meal Totals		**664**	**45**	**4**	**112**	**2**
3	Baked Potato	1 medium	164	4	0	37	4
	Beef Chili with Beans	1 cup	256	14	8	32	8
	Cheddar Cheese	1/2 cup (shredded)	231	14	19	1	0
	Sour Cream	1/4 cup	124	2	12	2	0
	Blueberry Juice	2 cups	224	0	0	56	0
	Meal Totals		**999**	**34**	**39**	**128**	**12**
4	Greek Yogurt	1 container (5.3 oz)	108	15	0	12	0
	Honey	4 TBSP	280	0	0	70	0
	Whey Protein Powder	1 scoop	104	20	0	6	0
	Meal Totals		**492**	**35**	**0**	**88**	**0**
5	Lean Beef Steak	6 ounces	232	40	8	0	0
	A-1 Steak Sauce	4 TBSP	48	0	0	12	0
	Quinoa	1 cup	224	8	4	39	5
	Green Beans	1 cup	36	2	0	7	3
	Bell Pepper	1/2 cup	24	1	0	5	1
	Meal Totals		**564**	**51**	**12**	**63**	**9**
6	Plum	1 medium	32	0	0	8	1
	Muscle Milk	2 scoops	338	32	18	12	0
	Meal Totals		**370**	**32**	**18**	**20**	**1**
	Daily Totals		**3987**	**254**	**99**	**520**	**35**

CHAPTER 3:
The Science Behind This Plan

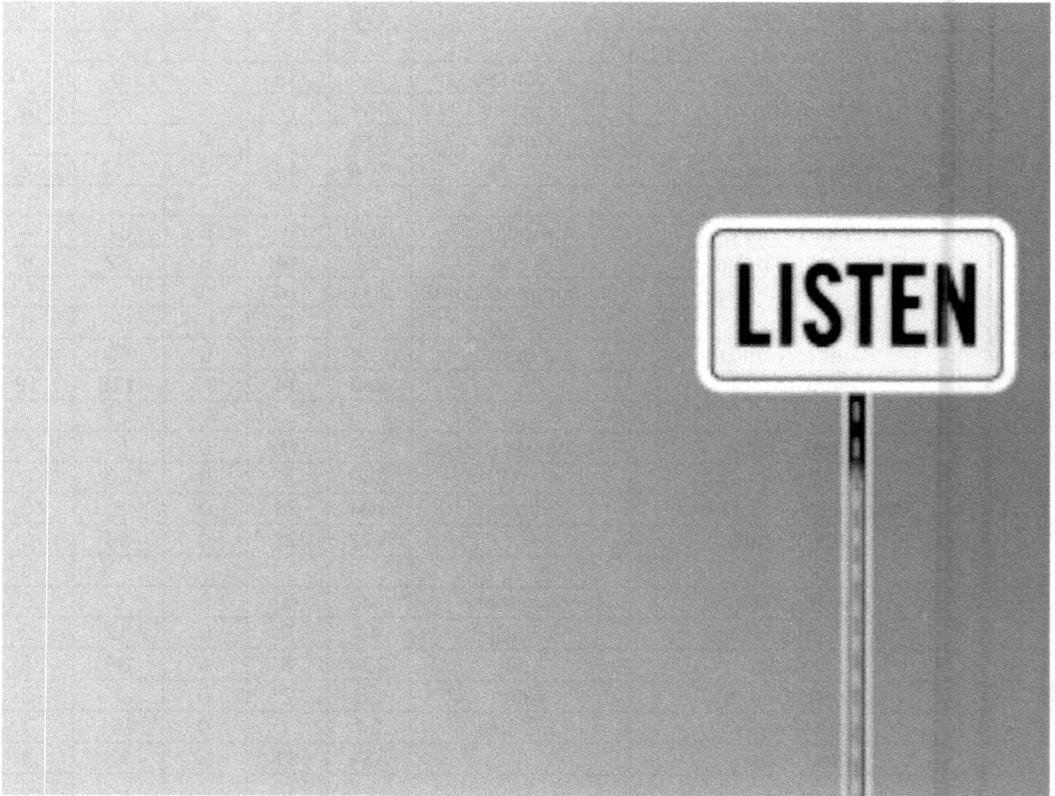

Now that you've read how well this plan has worked for others and you've seen the plan itself, you may be wondering what the science behind the plan is. Those answers are provided here. To make it more user-friendly, we have put it in an atypical format—it has all been done in bullet points. We did this for you: to save you time and to provide the greatest amount of information in the most concise manner possible. By reducing reading time, you save a few hours that could be used for exercising (hint, hint). Besides, you've already heard our stories—once upon a time, we were large as well but we researched the perfect diet, went on the diet and now we're full of vitality, vim and vigor. Enjoy this. The amount of information here is amazing.

THE COLD HARD FACTS OF WHERE WE ARE

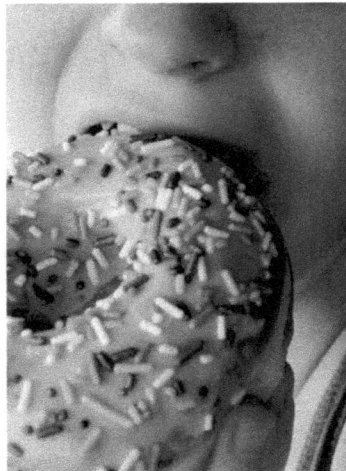

- We have approximately 300 million people in the United States and over a quarter of them are obese.
- Only 12% of individuals who go on a weight-loss program actually lose weight and only 2% of them will maintain their weight loss for over one year.
- It is estimated that about 400,000 Americans die each year as a result of being obese. (This statistic rivals those statistics associated with smoking).
- Taxpayers pay out approximately 75 billion dollars a year to cover medical costs related to obesity.
- In 2005, the government spent 440 million dollars on obesity-related research.

- About 10-15% of American children and 30% of the adult population are obese.
- There are almost seven billion people in the world and one third of them are suffering from malnutrition.
- We live in the most medically advanced country in the world; yet the statistical success rate of most medical weight loss programs is just about none.
- The success rate of helping someone lose weight is about 2%. That is incredible when you realize the success rate of curing cancer is about 40%.
- Our biological system interacts with our intrapsychic and social system to mold our behavior—if you want to control your eating behavior, you must pay attention not only to your body chemistry, but also to your psychological make-up and social environment.

HOW THIS IMPACTS YOU

- Obesity predisposes an individual to medical disorders such as heart disease, kidney disease, diabetes mellitus, high blood pressure, breathing disorders and greater risk during surgery.
- It has been scientifically estimated that if everybody were at their optimal weight, there would be twenty-five percent fewer cases of coronary heart disease in the USA.
- There are psychological as well as medical hazards associated with obesity:
  - Obese people are discriminated against with respect to employment, promotion and social acceptance.
  - Obese people are more likely to have low self-esteem and experience more anxiety, depression, loneliness and unhappiness.

ABOUT CALORIES:

- A **calorie** is a measure of heat and energy. Calories indicate the amount of energy provided by any particular food or drink.
    - Technically, a calorie is the amount of heat required to raise the temperature of one gram of water one degree centigrade.
- Basically, if more calories are consumed than are used in a normal day's activity, the excess is stored primarily as fat. Conversely, if more calories are burned than are consumed, weight is lost.
    - For example, if a person needs 2,000 calories a day to sustain his present body weight and consumes 2,500 calories, the extra 500 calories will be stored primarily as fat. If that individual continues to eat 500 calories more than needed each day for a period of seven days, he will gain one pound of weight.
    - Translated into simple terms: one pound of weight is equal to 3,500 calories.
- A male needs approximately 20 calories to maintain one pound of body weight.
- A female needs approximately 18 calories to maintain one pound of body weight.
- It is best to eat five or six times a day to maintain a constant blood glucose concentration level.

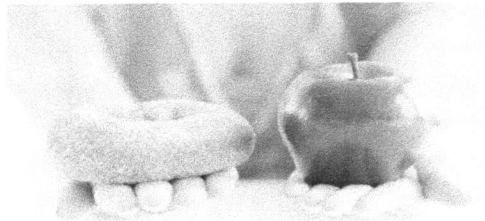

- Exercise will burn off calories, dampen your appetite, speed up your metabolism and ward off stress and anxiety.
- In order to control body weight, caloric intake and calorie expenditure must be systematically controlled. Deliberate voluntary weight control would be harder without adequate knowledge of the calorie content of food and beverages.
- A **nutrient** is any chemical substance present in food that provides the body with energy or with building materials required for normal metabolic function.
- It is not food that is the problem; it is the quantity and quality of food that is consumed that leads to problems.

ABOUT CARBOHYDRATES:

- **Carbohydrates** are the first of the three macronutrients your body needs. (A **macronutrient** is a nutrient your body needs in large amounts.)
- The primary purpose of carbohydrates is to supply the body with energy and/or calories.
- Carbohydrates are the principal source of energy for the muscles during exercise.
- Carbohydrates help regulate protein and fat metabolism; they are essential for the breakdown of free fatty acids within the liver.
- One gram of carbohydrate provides 4 calories.
- Most experts recommend that 50 to 60 percent of the total calories in a normal

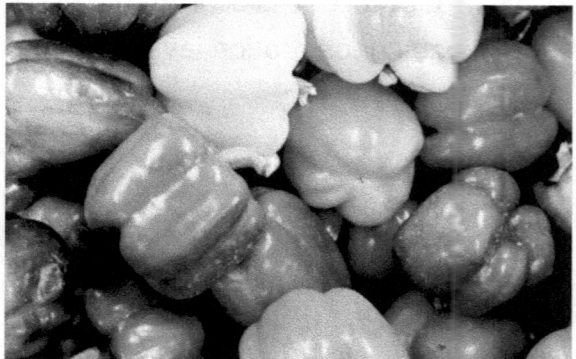

person's diet should come from carbohydrates.

- The bulk of our carbohydrate intake should be from the complex carbohydrates such as vegetables and pure grains but we need to ingest more simple carbohydrates as well, such as those found in fruits, milk and yogurt. All of these sources are vitamin-, mineral- and nutrient-rich, unlike man-made carbohydrates in most cases.
- There are "good" carbohydrates and "bad" carbohydrates.
    - "Good" carbohydrates are most anything grown from the Earth.
    - "Bad" carbohydrates are most anything made from Man.
- During digestion the body breaks carbohydrates into glucose and stores it in the muscles as glycogen.
- During exercise, the glycogen is converted back to glucose and is used for energy.
- The ability to sustain prolonged vigorous exercise is directly related to initial levels of muscle glycogen.
- Carbohydrate metabolism must be considered for development of muscle mass and strength.
- In order for muscle cells to absorb amino acids, a number of hormones must be present. It is important for muscle cells to absorb amino acids for the repairing and building of muscle tissue.
- One of the most growth-promoting hormones in the body is insulin, which is released whenever carbohydrates are eaten.
- Insulin's primary job is to regulate the glucose concentration in the blood.
- When carbohydrates are ingested, insulin is released by the body, which in turn stimulates cells to take up glucose.
- This release of insulin also has a potent anabolic (growth) effect.
- The insulin causes the muscle cells to absorb amino acids, thereby, stimulating muscle protein synthesis. This will aid in both the growth and repair of muscle tissues depleted by exercise, and enables a

person to have more energy because the body is in a state of repair, rather than disrepair.

- It has been well documented that eating protein and carbohydrates to promote insulin release results in about a 50% greater muscle protein synthesis than eating just protein.
- Sufficient dietary carbohydrate ingestion is needed in order to reduce the amount of catabolic stress hormones, such as cortisol and adrenaline.
- The Glycemic Index simply tells you how quickly a carbohydrate is converted to usable sugars right after you eat it.
    - Basically, it is how quickly your body can turn the carbohydrates you eat into energy.
    - Both high and low rated carbohydrates have a place in your diet.
    - When you need sustained energy, i.e., during a workout, you would want to eat a carbohydrate with a low rating.
    - When you need instant energy, say right after your workout for recuperative benefits, a higher-rated carbohydrate would be better.

Glycemic Index Values for Carbohydrates

Ranging From 39 to 55

Food	Glycemic Index Rating	Food Category
Apple juice (unsweetened)	42	fruit
Apple	39	fruit
Apple, dried	39	fruit
Apricots, dried	41	fruit
Baked beans	46	starch
Banana bread	46	starch
Black beans, boiled	41	starch
Black-eyed peas, canned	40	starch
Breads		
100% whole wheat	43	starch
pumpernickel, whole grain	41	starch
Sourdough	40	starch
Cereals		
Kellogg's All-Bran, extra fiber	40	starch
Bran-Bud's w/ psyllium	40	starch
Oatmeal w/ water	40	starch
Oat bran	40	starch
Special K	43	starch
Bulgar, cooked	40	starch
Butterbeans (lima), boiled	43	starch
Cherries	40	fruit
Chocolate bar	50	sugar
Custard	40	starch
Fruit toast, pure	50	sugar
Grapefruit juice, unsweetened	40	fruit
Grapefruit, raw	40	fruit
Ice milk, vanilla	50	dairy, sugar
Kidney beans		
Red, boiled	40	starch
Red, canned & dried	40	starch
Kiwi, medium & raw	40	fruit
Lactose, pure	40	sugar
Lentil soup	40	starch
Lima beans, baby & frozen	40	starch

Food	Glycemic Index Rating	Food Category
Milk		
Chocolate flavored, 1%	50	dairy, sugar
Skim	40	dairy
Whole	40	dairy
Muffins		
Apple-cinnamon	50	starch
Chocolate butterscotch (low fat)	50	starch
Navy beans, boiled	40	starch
Orange, navel	50	fruit
PastaCappelletti, cooked	50	starch
Fettuccine, cooked	50	starch
Linguine, thick & cooked	50	starch
Pasta		
Macaroni, cooked	50	starch
Ravioli, meat-filled & cooked	50	starch
Spaghetti, white & cooked	50	starch
Spaghetti, whole wheat & cooked	50	starch
Star pastina, cooked	50	starch
Tortellini, cheese & cooked	50	starch
Vermicelli, cooked	50	starch
Peaches		
Canned, light syrup	50	fruit
Canned, natural juice	50	fruit
Fresh, 1 medium	50	fruit
Pears		
Canned in pear juice	50	fruit
Fresh	50	fruit
Peas		
Dried, boiled	40	fruit
Green, fresh, frozen, boiled	40	fruit
Pinto beans		
Canned	40	starch
Soaked, boiled	40	starch
Plums	50	fruit
Potato chips, plain	50	starch
Sweet potatoes, peeled, boiled	50	starch
Pound cake	50	starch
Rice bran	40	starch
Rice		
Converted, Uncle Ben's	40	starch
Parboiled	40	starch

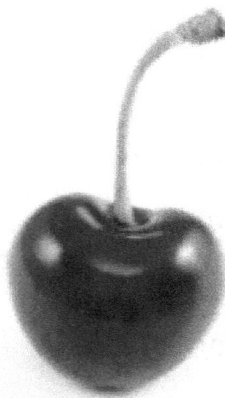

Food	Glycemic Index Rating	Food Category
Soybeans, boiled	40	starch
Soy milk	40	dairy
Split peas, yellow & boiled	40	starch
Sponge cake, plain	40	starch
Stone wheat thins	40	starch
Tomato soup, canned	40	starch
Twix chocolate caramel cookie	50	starch
Yam, boiled	51	starch
Yogurt non-fat		
Fruit flavored, artificial sweetener	50	dairy
Fruit flavored, with sugar	50	dairy
Plain, artificial sweetener	50	dairy

Glycemic Index Values for Carbohydrates

Ranging From 56 to 75

Food	Glycemic Index Rating	Food Category
Angel food cake	60	starch
Apricot jam, no added sugar	60	fruit
Apricot, canned, light syrup	60	fruit
Apricot, fresh	60	fruit
Banana, raw	60	fruit
Beets, canned & drained	60	vegetable
Blackbean soup	63	starch
Breads		
Hamburger bun	64	starch
Light deli, (American) rye	62	starch
Melba toast	60	starch
Pita bread, whole-wheat	60	starch
Rye	60	starch
Soy dough rye, Arnold's	60	starch
Whole-wheat	60	starch
Cereals		
Cream of Wheat, cooked	65	starch
Frosted Flakes, Kellogg's	74	starch
Grape Nuts, Post	70	starch
Just Right	70	starch
Life, Quaker	70	starch
Mini Wheats, whole-wheat	70	starch
Muesli, natural muesli	72	starch
Multi-bran Chex, General Mills	71	starch
Oats, 1 minute, Quaker	70	starch
Puffed wheat, Quaker	62	starch
Shredded wheat, spoon size	64	starch
Smacks, Kellogg's	60	starch
Cantaloupe, raw	70	fruit
Coca-Cola	70	sugar
Corn, canned & drained	65	starch
Cornmeal, from mix, cooked	68	starch
Couscous, cooked	65	starch
Croissant, medium	70	starch
Fanta	70	sugar
Flame	73	sugar

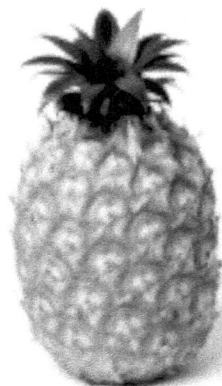

Food	Glycemic Index Rating	Food Category
Fruit cocktail, natural juice	70	fruit
Granola bars, Quaker chewy	72	starch
Green pea soup	63	starch
Honey	70	sugar
Ice cream, 10% fat, vanilla	72	dairy, sugar
Kudos, granola bars (whole-grain)	73	starch
Macaroni & cheese dinner, Kraft packaged	73	starch
Mango	68	fruit
Muffins		
Low fat from mix	70	starch
Low fat from mix	72	starch
Blueberry	68	starch
Oat bran	61	starch
Oat Bran, raw	63	starch
Papaya	60	fruit
Pasta		
Gnocchi, cooked	60	starch
Linguine, cooked	60	starch
Pastry, flaky	65	starch
Pea soup, split with hand	68	starch
Peaches, canned, heavy syrup	71	fruit
Pineapple, fresh	70	fruit
Pizza, cheese & tomato	70	starch
Popcorn, light, microwave	60	starch
Potatoes		
New, canned, drained	70	starch
New, peeled, boiled	70	starch
White-skinned, mashed	69	starch
White-skinned, peeled, boiled	70	starch
Raisins	72	fruit
Rice vermicelli, cooked	70	starch
Rice		
Brown	65	starch
Basmati, white, boiled	65	starch
Long-grain, white	65	starch
Shortbread cookies	60	starch
Skittles, original, fruit, bite size candy	70	sugar
Social tea biscuits, Nabisco	60	starch
Split pea soup	60	starch
Sucrose	73	sugar
Taco shells	65	starch

Glycemic Index Values for Carbohydrates

Ranging From 76 to 100

Food	Glycemic Index Rating	Food Category
Bagel	80	starch
Breads		
Kaiser roll	80	starch
Dark rye, black bread	80	starch
Dark rye, Schinkenbrot	80	starch
French baguette	80	starch
White	80	starch
Cereals		
Bran Flakes, Post	83	starch
Cheerios, General Mills	82	starch
Cocoa Krispies, Kellogg's	85	starch
Corn bran, Quaker crunchy	80	starch
Corn Chex	81	starch
Corn Flakes, Kellogg's	81	starch
Cream of Wheat, instant	80	starch
Crispix, Kellogg's	84	starch
Golden Grahams, General Mills	81	starch
Grape Nut Flakes, Post	80	starch
Raisin Bran, Kellogg's	83	starch
Rice Chex	83	starch
Rice Krispies, Kellogg's	85	starch
Shredded Wheat, Post	81	starch
Total, General Mills	80	starch
Weetabix	80	starch
Corn chips	80	starch
Crispbread	81	starch
Dates, dried	80	fruit
Doughnut with cinnamon & sugar	90	starch
Fava beans, frozen, boiled	82	starch
Gatorade Sports Drink	90	sugar
Glucose powder	91	sugar
Graham crackers	85	starch
Jelly beans	90	sugar
Maltose (maltodextrin), pure	90	sugar
Mullet, cooked	80	starch
Parsnips, boiled	82	starch

Food	Glycemic Index Rating	Food Category
Potatoes		
Instant mashed, carnation foods	90	starch
Red-skinned, baked in oven, no fat	90	starch
Red-skinned, mashed	91	starch
Red-skinned, microwaved	91	starch
Red-skinned, peeled, boiled	90	starch
Baked in oven, no fat	90	starch
White-skinned, with skin, microwaved	91	starch
Premium Saltine Crackers	90	starch
Pretzels	90	starch
Rice Cakes, plain	91	starch
Rice		
Instant, cooked	90	starch
Short-grain, white (sticky)	90	starch
Rutabaga, peeled, boiled	90	starch
Vanilla Wafers	90	starch
Waffles, plain, frozen	90	starch
Water Cracker, Carrs	91	starch
Watermelon	90	fruit

ABOUT THAT SUGAR YOU LOVE SO MUCH

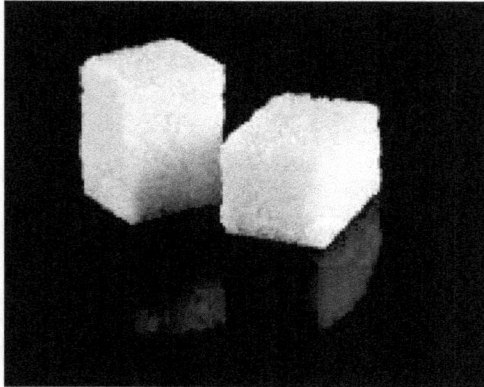

Think of it as poison. We're not talking about the carbohydrates God put on earth for us, like vegetables, fruits and real whole grains. We're talking about the ones man either made or genetically altered, like candy bars, crackers, sodas, genetically modified wheat, etc. You know—the manufactured things we made so that we could sit them on the shelf for nine months without any sign of deterioration.

There are two main reasons to think of sugar as poison. The first is to help you break your psychological addiction to it. Go ahead and admit it. There are foods you just "have to have." In reality, you can live without them but you are tricked into thinking you can't. The grip they have on you is killing you but all you see is the sweetness. The second reason to think it is poison is because it *is* poison. If you don't believe us, consider this:

- Sugar increases total body inflammation.
- Sugar causes cardiovascular diseases.
- Sugar can increase one's cholesterol.
- Sugar can cause diabetes.

- Sugar can cause cancer and speed it up like gasoline on a fire.
- Sugar can cause obesity.
- Sugar can weaken the eyesight.
- Sugar can cause a decrease in growth hormone production.
- Sugar can cause food allergies.
- Sugar can cause hyperactivity.
- Sugar rushes can cause drowsiness and decreases in energy after the rush ends.
- Sugar can cause a decrease in protein absorption.
- Sugar can cause eczema.
- Sugar can cause the structure of DNA to change.
- Sugar can cause anxiety disorders.
- Sugar can cause osteoporosis.
- Sugar can cause cramping.
- Sugar can cause joint pain.
- Sugar feeds yeast infections.
- Sugar interferes with the body's ability to rid itself of bacteria by lowering white blood cell counts.
- Sugar impairs the immune system, making one more susceptible to illnesses.
- Sugar can cause deeper facial wrinkles.
- Sugar can cause saggy skin.
- Sugar can cause puffiness in the face.
- Sugar can cause dark circles around the eyes.
- Sugar can exacerbate acne.
- Sugar can decrease the beneficial cholesterol, HDL's.
- Sugar can cause severe periodontal disease.
- Sugar can upset the mineral balance.
- Sugar can cause a copper deficiency.

- Sugar can cause a chromium deficiency.
- Sugar can cause an increase in triglycerides.
- Sugar can impair nutrient absorption and digestion.
- Sugar can cause grey hair.

There are more but we've spent enough time on sugar. The fact is experts recommend we ingest no more than 6 (not 6 as in you have to max it out, that's no more than 6 but ideally lower than that) tablespoons of sugar a day. The average American takes in twenty two-tablespoons a day which totals to 168 pounds a year.

If you want better skin, better vitality, more consistent energy and a healthier body, cut out that sugar. It seems beautiful, fun and sweet, but it's all been a lie. It's poison.

ABOUT FIBER:

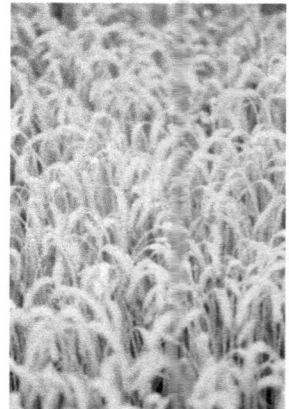

- Fiber has two forms: **insoluble** and **soluble**.
    - Soluble fiber forms a gel when mixed with liquid, while water-soluble fiber does not.
    - Soluble fiber lowers cholesterol, as well as blood sugar levels in people with diabetes. Some researchers have found that increasing fiber decreases the body's need for insulin.
    - Water-soluble fiber comes most from whole wheat products which increase the bulk in the digestive track and enhances elimination.
- The typical American consumes approximately 18 to 20 grams of fiber a day.
- The National Cancer Institute recommends consuming 25 to 40 grams of fiber a day.

ABOUT FATS:

- **Fats** are the second of the three macronutrients that your body needs.
- Fats supply the body with energy and are a source of vitamins A, D, E and K.
- They provide protection and support for organs such as the heart, kidneys and liver.
- Fats insulate the body from environmental temperature changes and help make calcium available to body tissues, particularly the bones and teeth.
- There are two types of fatty acids: **saturated** and **unsaturated**.
  - Foods that are high in saturated fats include fatty meats, coconut oil and chocolate, dairy products (cheese, cream and butter) and animal fats (lard, tallow and suet).
  - Unsaturated fats are mostly found in vegetable sources.
- Saturated fats are not heart-healthy since they are most known for raising your LDL cholesterol ("bad" cholesterol).
- HDLs are good fats and LDLs are the bad fats.
- HDLs will actually "eat" the LDL's in your body.
- An increase in LDLs can predispose you to arteriosclerosis, which is the occlusion of the artery.
- *TRANS FATS*:
  - Trans fats are hydrogenated vegetable fats.
  - They raise LDL levels ("bad" cholesterol) and lowers HDL levels ("good" cholesterol). They clog arteries and increase the risk of stroking or developing heart disease.

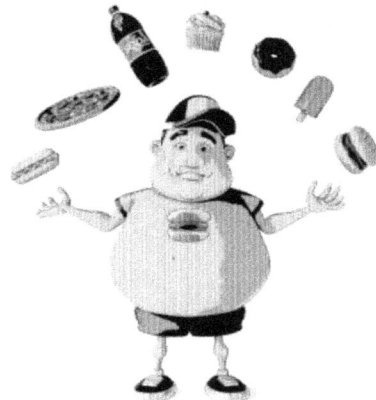

- Trans fats are used by food processors because they allow longer shelf-life and give food desirable taste, shape and texturing.
- The majority of trans fats can be found in shortenings, stick (or hard) margarine, cookies, crackers, snack foods, fried foods (including fried fast food), doughnuts, pastries, baked goods and other processed foods made with or fried in partially hydrogenated oils.

ABOUT PROTEINS:

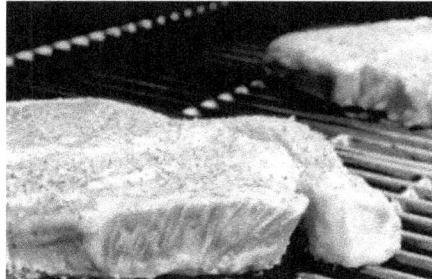

- **Proteins** are the third and final macronutrient your body needs.
- Proteins make up more than twenty percent of our total body weight.
- Next to water, protein is the most plentiful substance in the body.
- Protein is the major source of building material for muscles, hair, teeth, eyes, nails and scar tissue.
- Protein is also necessary for the formation of hormones.
- Protein is used to form enzymes, substances that are necessary for basic life functions, and antibodies, which help fight invading antigens.
- Protein also helps prevent blood and tissues from becoming either too acidic or too alkaline and helps maintain the body's water balance.
- Generally, protein provides approximately 10 to 15 percent of energy during aerobic exercise.
- The body requires twenty-two amino acids in a specific arrangement to produce human protein.
  - Unfortunately, the body can only produce fourteen of these amino acids. These are called "non-essential amino acids".
    - The other eight amino acids, which are referred to as the "essential amino acids", must be supplied by the diet.
- In order for the body to properly synthesize protein, all twenty-two amino acids must be present simultaneously and in the proper proportions.
- If even one of the "essential amino acids" is missing, even temporarily,

protein synthesis will be significantly compromised or stop completely.

- Not all foods contain all the essential amino acids.
- The ones that do are called "complete proteins"; the foods that don't are called "incomplete proteins".
- Most animal proteins and dietary products—meat, milk, milk products, fish, poultry and eggs—are "complete proteins".
- Most plant proteins–grains, beans, vegetables and fruits—are "incomplete proteins".
- A complete protein meal can be constructed from incomplete proteins, but the foods must be combined carefully to ensure that the deficient amino acids will be adequately balanced by other amino acids.
- Just as too little protein is bad for you, too much protein can present health problems.
  - Too much protein can put a strain on the liver and kidneys.
  - Some protein-rich foods are high in nucleic acids, which when broken down are converted into uric acid.
  - Too much uric acid in the blood can lead to gout.
  - Too much protein can also lead to osteoporosis (thinning of the bones) and promote the loss of calcium in the bones through urine.

ABOUT WATER:

- Water is the most essential nutrient.
- We can survive weeks without food but only a few days without water.
- Approximately 60% of the body and 70% of the brain are composed of water.
- Just about every biological process, including digestion, absorption, circulation and excretion, is contingent upon water.
- Water is the main component of the blood.
- Water is the primary transporter of nutrients throughout the body and is essential for all building functions.
- Water helps maintain normal body temperature and is paramount in carrying waste products out of the body.
- The average individual needs approximately eight to ten glasses of water a day, or about two quarts. (You may not be the average.)
- How much water you actually need depends on your weight, level of activity, the temperature and humidity of your environment, and your diet.
- Approximately two thirds of our daily water intake comes from beverages and one third from food.
- Dehydration can impair mental and physical performance by up to 25%.

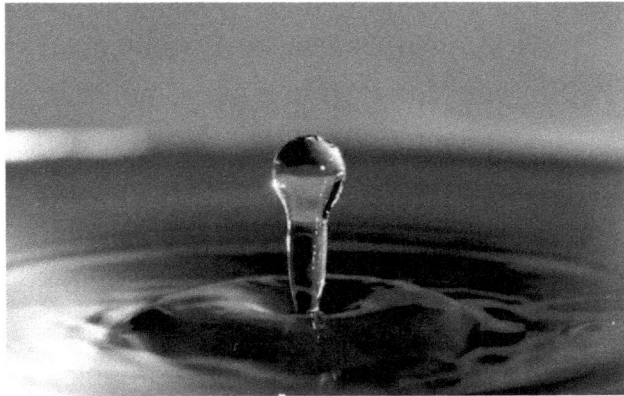

ABOUT VITAMINS:

- **Vitamins** are indispensable organic compounds.
- Vitamins perform various bodily functions that promote growth, reproduction and maintain health.
- Vitamins are usually differentiated as being water-soluble or fat-soluble.
    - Fat-soluble vitamins, A, D, E and K, are stored by the body and do not need to be consumed on a daily basis.
    - Deficiencies of fat-soluble vitamins are rare.
    - Excessive consumption of these vitamins, especially A and D, can be toxic.
    - Water-soluble vitamins, B-complex vitamins, vitamins C and the compounds termed "bioflavonoids" are not stored in fat and therefore, must be consumed frequently.
    - Vitamin deficiencies can cause malfunction of bodily functions and can lead to such ailments as heart disease and glandular and nervous disorders.
- If you eat a balanced diet that includes food from all major groups, there may not be a need to take vitamin supplements. The food you eat should provide you with all the vitamins and minerals you need.
- You should be getting a minimum of five or more servings of fruits and vegetables a day.
- Taking a good multi-vitamin may be a sound insurance plan to protect against vitamin deficiency.
- Quality vitamin supplements are safe, inexpensive and effective in preventing vitamin or mineral deficiencies.

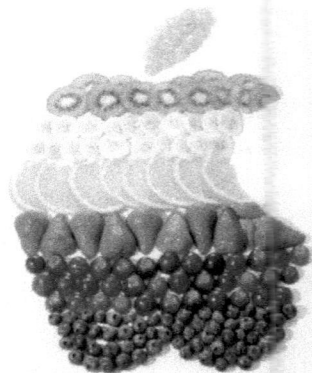

ABOUT MINERALS:

- **Minerals** are essential for metabolic functions such as regulating the release of energy.
- Minerals are important for muscle contraction, nerve transmission, protein synthesis, development of hormones, and formation of teeth, bones and hemoglobin.
    - Other functions of minerals include balancing water and acidity.
- A l of the minerals needed by the human body must be supplied by an individual's diet.
- Generally, a well-balanced diet of animal and vegetable origin will furnish more than adequate minerals.
- There are six major minerals: calcium, phosphorous, magnesium, potassium, sodium and chloride.
- There are fourteen trace minerals: chromium, cobalt, copper, fluorine, iodine, iron, manganese, molybdenum, nickel, selenium, silicon, tin, vanadium and zinc.
- A mineral deficiency often results in an illness, which may be remedied by the addition of the missing mineral in the diet.

Vitamins and Minerals Chart

Nutrient	Functions in the Body/Benefits	Dietary Sources	Maximum Daily Dose/Toxicities
Vitamin A Retinol, beta-carotene and various other carotenoids	Helps maintain good vision (necessary for night vision), resistance to infections, sand supports growth and repair of body tissues. Also maintains integrity of white and red blood cells, and epithelial lining. Used to treat acne.	Milk, eggs, meat, fish liver oils. Beta-carotene and other carotenoids are found in: Green leafy vegetables - kale, spinach, broccoli, collard greens, parsley, turnip greens, escarole. Yellow vegetables - carrots, sweet potatoes, winter squash, pumpkin. Yellow and orange fruits - mango, cantaloupe, papaya, apricots.	5,000 IU is best (in beta-carotene form); max/day 20,000 IU. Stop immediately if you experience nausea and vomiting, blurred vision, or bone pain. A harmless orange coloring of the palms and the face may develop with excessive intake of beta-carotene.
Vitamin D	Regulates absorption of calcium and phosphorus for bone health.	Formed in skin when exposed to sunlight. Also found in dairy products, egg yolks, fish liver oils, tuna, mackerel, herring, sardines, oysters, yeast.	800-1,200 IU. Don't give kids more than 1000 IU; excess doses may result in hypercalcemia, which can damage the kidneys and weaken the bones.

Vitamin E Tocopherols, tocotrienols	Antioxidant. Helps maintain cell membranes and red blood cell integrity. Protects vitamin A and fatty acids from oxidation. Used to treat anemia and may help manage claudication (cramping pain caused by low blood supply to affected muscles).	Found primarily in vegetable oils, but also butter, avocados, eggs, nuts, whole grain cereals, wheat germ. Fat malabsorption can lead to vitamin E deficiency.	1,200 IU Such high amounts may interfere with vitamin K activity and increase the risk of uncontrolled bleeding. Important to know what type of tocopherol you're getting in a supplement.
Vitamin K	Helps make factors that promote blood clotting. Used to treat hemorrhagic disorders.	Gut produces some. Diet generally supplies remaining need. Some stored in liver. Green, leafy vegetables are the best source, followed by liver and other animal foods. Fat malabsorption can lead to vitamin K deficiency.	80 mcg Phylloquinone is essentially non-toxic; otherwise, take care with use, especially in children.

Vitamin B1 Thiamin	Helps metabolize carbohydrates, maintain appetite and normal digestion. Essential for nervous tissue function. May be part of a regimen to offset mitochondrial toxicity.	Found in many foods: whole grain cereals, peas, beans, peanuts, legumes, brewer's yeast, wheat germ. Alcohol, malnutrition, diarrhea, & malabsorption contribute to vitamin B1 deficiency.	Very safe. One German study used 320 mg/day for neuropathy with no side effects.
Vitamin B2 Riboflavin	Helps body break down amino acids, regulates energy, growth, hormones, and formation of red blood cells. Supports cellular breathing. Prevents red, cracked lips and burning tongue. May help with high lactate or lactic acidosis.	Egg whites, greens, lean meat, fish, wheat germ, milk.	Very safe. 200 mg a day is probably excreted. B vitamin complexes can include from 50 -100 mg/day of riboflavin. Standard multivitamins contain 3 mg.

Vitamin B3 Niacin, nicotiric acid, niacinamide	Important for fat synthesis, protein and carbohydrate breakdown, tissue respiration, health of skin, tongue, digestive system. Higher doses may help manage cholesterol.	Yeast, lean meat, chicken, salmon, tuna, legumes, whole grain cereals, peanuts.	Niacin: Standard formulations of multivitamins can contain 20-30 mg. B-complex supplements contain 100 mg, some have up to 200 mg. Supplementation at this dose can cause flushing or itching. Higher doses are sometimes used to treat high LDL cholesterol but can cause liver damage, high blood sugar, vomiting, diarrhea, and low blood pressure. This should be done only with a physician's supervision. Niacinamide: A non-itchy, no-flush form of B3. 250 mg is typically a safe daily dose. Higher doses may be tolerated. Niacinamide isn't associated with causing low blood pressure and doesn't work to treat high cholesterol.

Vitamin B5	Helps body metabolize carbohydrates, fats, and make steroids. Offsets deficiency-related dermatitis and "burning foot" syndrome.	Eggs, chicken, avocados, soybeans, whole grains. Deficiency is uncommon due to its widespread availability in foods.	10 mg included in most supplements. B vitamin complexes can include from 5-75 mg.
Vitamin B6 Pyridoxine, pyridoxal, other forms	Various classes of enzymes (e.g., aminotransferases) depend on B6 for their activity. Often prescribed to offset the depletion caused by the TB drug, Isoniazid.	Chicken, fish, pork, liver, eggs, rice, soybeans, oats, whole wheat, peanuts, walnuts, bananas, avocados.	250 mg; more than this may worsen or cause neuropathy; high doses probably are best taken with a B-complex; more data needed.
Vitamin B12 Cobalamin	Red blood cell health and development, treat pernicious anemia, used in management of neuropathy.	Liver, kidney, dairy, eggs. B12 is synthesized by intestinal bacteria. Many people use acidophilus supplements to help maintain intestinal flora.	1,000 mcg; non-toxic. Absorption of B12 is more complicated than other B vitamins. The body can make and recycle some B12 from what comes in, but absorption of this vitamin can be disrupted in both the stomach and the intestines. If absorption is a problem, B12 may need to be administered by injection.

Biotin	Deficiency can result in hair loss, dermatitis. Biotinyl proteins are critical for fat, carbohydrate and amino acid metabolism.	Yeast, liver, kidney, eggs, milk, fish, nuts.	No known toxicity. B complex vitamins can contain from 30 to 100 mcg of biotin.
Vitamin C (ascorbic acid; also may be found bound to minerals such as in calcium ascorbate)	Essential element in collagen formation. Important for wound healing, bone fractures, and resistance to infections. Strengthens blood vessels. Helps body absorb non-heme iron when the two are ingested together.	Abundant in most fresh fruits (esp. citrus) and vegetables.	No toxic limit. However, if you take too much too fast (greater than a 2,000 mg dose), you may have diarrhea. Ascorbate forms are easier on the intestine; raise dosage slowly.
Folic acid Folate folacin	Essential for blood cell formation, protein metabolism, and prevention of neural tube defects.	Green leafy vegetables, liver, kidney, yeast, orange juice, fortified grain products, beans.	Very non-toxic, particularly if taken with adequate B12. High dosages may mask a vitamin B12 deficiency.
Boron	Bone health, prevention of osteoporosis, reduces magnesium excretion.	Fruits, vegetables.	3 mg/day is a suggested dose; take with multi containing manganese, calcium and riboflavin.

Calcium	Necessary for strong bone structure, teeth, muscle tissue. Regulates heartbeat, nerve function. Plasma levels affected by thyroid, parathyroid glands.	Green leafy vegetables, fortified orange juice, dairy products. Sardines, salmon with bones, tofu. Alcohol, soda (colas) & caffeine deplete calcium stores in body. Need vitamin D to make use of calcium in the body.	Overdose unlikely unless you are magnesium deficient; iron & zinc absorption may be impaired with high calcium intake. High intake may cause constipation. Daily intake need varies depending on age, gender, and health. Talk with your doctor about the right dose for you.
Chromium	Glucose metabolism. Deficiency results in glucose intolerance.	Brewer's yeast, whole grain cereals, nuts, black pepper, thyme, meat, cheese.	300 mcg; around 1,000 mcg/day for certain conditions is typically safe.
Copper	Supports healthy bones, muscles, and blood vessels. Assists in iron absorption.	Liver, legumes, nuts, seeds, raisins, whole grains, shellfish, shrimp.	5 mg; avoid if you have hemochromatosis or Wilson's disease; 10 mg will cause nausea; Upper Limit = 10,000 mcg/day.
Iodine	Essential component of thyroid hormones that regulate tissue growth and cell activity.	Iodized salt, seafood, bread, milk, cheese.	150 - 250 mcg. High doses are not usually a problem unless you have hyperthyroid disease.

Iron	Supports red blood cell health through formation of hemoglobin in blood and myoglobin, which supplies oxygen to muscles. Key for menstruating women in preventing iron-deficiency anemia.	Red meats, Liver, poultry, fish, beans, peas, dried apricots, blackstrap molasses. Certain foods, like grains, contain phytates, which may inhibit iron absorption. Vegetarians may not get enough iron from their diet.	30 mg/day max; avoid extra if you have liver disease or hemochromatosis; excess can cause bloody diarrhea, vomiting, acidosis, darkened stools, abdominal pain. Non-heme (plant sources) iron absorbed poorly.
Magnesium	Important for parathyroid hormone release, muscle contraction, bone formation, blood pressure control. Deficiency occurs with malabsorption/ alcoholism/ kidney disorders and may result in lowered calcium & potassium levels.	Nuts, legumes, unmilled grains, beans, green leafy vegetables, avocados, bananas.	Trace element supplements can contain from 100-500 mg. Higher doses (up to 1000 mg) may also have benefit, but more data needed. Supplementation may be problematic if you have kidney trouble; first signs of excess are low blood pressure, nausea and vomiting.
Manganese	Involved in the formation of bone, as well as in enzymes involved in amino acid, cholesterol, and carbohydrate metabolism.	Nuts, whole grain cereals, beans, rice, dried fruits, green leafy vegetables.	10 mg. Higher doses can interfere with iron absorption.

Molybdenum	Important in a variety of enzyme systems (e.g., oxidases). Mobilization of iron from storage, growth and development.	Milk, beans, whole grain breads and cereals, nuts, legumes (depending on soil content).	75-250 mcg it's not clear what the limit is but this is generally a safe and adequate range. A high incidence of gout-like syndrome has been associated with dietary intakes of 10-15 mg/day.
Phosphate	Bone health. See calcium entry. Maintains acid-base balance.	Don't supplement if you eat meat or drink sodas. Abundant in all animal foods: meat, fish, poultry, eggs, and milk.	500 mg. High consumption of phosphate may affect calcium levels.
Potassium (electrolyte)	Along with sodium and chloride, referred to as electrolytes. Maintains fluid balance, blood pressure, cell integrity, muscle contractions, and nerve impulse transmission. Sodium/potassium ratios out of balance result in muscle and heart weakness, diarrhea.	Fruits and juices (a banana has about 450 mg), green leafy vegetables, meats.	2,000 mg. High doses are used in people with kidney disease; excessive doses can be problematic.

Selenium	Antioxidant properties protect body tissues against oxidative damage caused by radiation, pollution and normal body reactions. Red blood cell health. Deficiency results in growth failure, and hepatic necrosis.	Seafood, kidney, liver, selected grains. Keshan's syndrome occurs in regions with selenium-depleted soils.	600 mcg max; 200-400 mcg per day is more than enough; reduce dose if you get a "garlic" breath/ taste.
Zinc	Maintaining immune function; wound repair. Deficiency results in anorexia, growth retardation, lowered testosterone levels, hair loss, and impaired taste.	Meat, liver, eggs, seafood (oysters), whole grains (but the form is less absorbable).	A total daily intake of 40 mg. Be sure to take copper if taking 50-150 mg is a maximum dose. Be sure to take copper if taking this amount and only under guidance.

IU = International Units; mg = milligrams; mcg = micrograms; g = grams. (Note: 1,000 mg = 1 gram)

Compiled by George Carter, Jen Curry & Anya Romanowski, MS, RD, CDN AIDS Community Research Initiative of America (ACRIA), Spring 2002

ABOUT SERVING SIZES:

- A US Department of Agriculture study concluded that over 30% of consumers do not use or understand nutrition information available to them on food packages.
- The information that you learn from the rest of the Nutrition Facts label depends on the serving size.
- It is important that you pay attention to the serving size, including the number of servings in the package and compare it to how much you actually eat.
- For example, if there is 50 calories in one serving and you eat four servings, you have taken in 200 calories, (50 X 4 = 200), and quadruple the fat, protein, etc. that you have eaten.
- When you start checking labels you may be surprised how small some serving sizes actually are. For instance, some granola type cereals are a little as 1/4 cup serving!

Serving Sizes   **Everyday Objects**

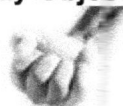

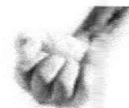

1 cup of cereal = a fist

1/2 cup of cooked rice, pasta, or potato = 1/2 baseball

1 baked potato = a fist

1 medium fruit = a baseball

1/2 cup of fresh fruit = 1/2 baseball

1 1/2 ounces of low-fat or fat-free cheese = 4 stacked dice

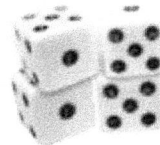

1/2 cup of ice cream = 1/2 baseball

2 tablespoons of peanut butter = a ping-pong ball

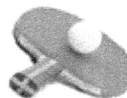

ABOUT LABEL READING:

- The Nutrition Facts food label contains information about calories, fat content, amount and types of carbohydrates and amount of protein.
- The % Daily Value shows how a food fits into a 2,000 calorie/day diet.
- The % Daily Value is probably the least important stat on the food label because it would have to be modified to meet each individual's specific case and needs.
- Right below the Amount Per Serving label you will see a Calories label. What this tells you is how many calories are in one serving.
- If the item is too calorie dense to fit into your nutrition place, you can stop reading right there.
- Calorie from Fat: This label tells you how many calories come from fat.
- Total Fat: This label shows you the amount of fat in one serving in grams.
    - There are 9 calories in one gram of fat.
- Right under Total Fat is Saturated Fat.
    - The accepted wisdom is to keep saturated fat down to less than 20

grams per day or no more than 10 percent of your total calories.

- Under the Saturated Fat label is Trans Fat.
  - This number should always be close to zero no matter how much fat you eat in a day.
- The next entry on the food label is Cholesterol.
- The United States Department of Agriculture recommends that most people should consume less than 200 mg of cholesterol a day.
  - The average American man consumes 360 mg of cholesterol a day.
  - The average American woman consumes between 220 mg and 260 mg.
- The next important ingredient on the food label is Sodium.
- Next on the food label is Total Carbohydrates.
  - There are 4 calories in one gram of carbohydrate.
- Under Total Carbohydrate you will see Sugars.
  - Sugars are simple carbohydrates.
- Not all Nutrition Facts labels contain a label for fiber.
- Next on the food label is Protein.
  - There are 4 calories in one gram of protein.
- The next section of the Nutrition Facts food label shows the vitamin content of the product.
- An ingredient list must be presented on all prepackaged products.
- The ingredient list, in many ways, is your best source of information.
- Contents are listed in descending order by weight, so the first two ingredients are usually the most prominent and important.
  - If the first ingredient is sugar (especially high fructose corn syrup) or enriched wheat flour (aka white flour), consider putting the package back on the shelf.
- All of the following are different terms for added sugar: brown sugar,

molasses, beet sugar, honey, cane juice, turbinado, maple syrup, corn syrup, dextrose, fructose, maltose, barley malt and fruit juice concentrate.

- Sugar alcohols, such as maltitol, xylitol and sorbitol can also have an impact on blood glucose levels.

- When reading the ingredient list you may see the word hydrogenated: hydrogenated and partially hydrogenated fats are dangerous in that they can cause atherosclerosis and high blood pressure.

ABOUT LABEL CLAIMS:

- Another aspect of food labeling is label claim.
- Here are some rules about some of those labels:

  - Free – A product contains no amount of, or only a trivial amount of, one of the following compounds: fat, saturated fat, cholesterol, sodium, sugars and calories. You may also see free foods labeled "without," "no" and "zero." These are synonyms for "free."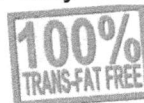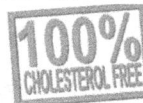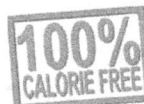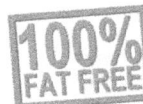

  - Calorie-Free – Fewer than 5 calories per serving.
  - Sugar-Free – Less than .5 grams per serving.
  - Fat-Free – Less than .5 grams per serving. Usually fat-free products have added sugar to make the food taste more palatable.
  - Low Fat – 3 grams or less per serving...that is 27 calories from fat.
  - Low Saturated Fat – 1 gram or less per serving.
  - Low Sodium – 140 milligrams or less per serving.
  - Very Low Sodium – 35 milligrams or less per serving.
  - Low Cholesterol – 20 milligrams or less and 2 grams or less of saturated fat per serving.
  - Low Calorie – 40 calories or less per serving.

- Lean and Extra Lean – These terms can be used to describe the fat content of meat, poultry, seafood and game meats.
  - Lean – Less than 10 grams of fat, 4.5 or less of saturated fat and less than 95 milligrams of cholesterol per serving and per 100 grams.
  - Extra Lean – Less than 5 grams of fat, less than 2 grams of saturated fat and less than 95 milligrams cholesterol per serving and per 100 grams.
- High – This term can be used if the food contains 20 percent or more of the daily value for a particular nutrient in a serving.
- Good Source – These terms mean that one serving of a food contains 10-19 percent of the Daily Value for a particular nutrient.
- Reduced – This term means that a nutritionally altered product contains at least 25 percent less of a nutrient or calories as compared to the regular or reference product. However, a reduced claim can't be made in a product if its reference food already meets the requirement for a low claim.
- Less – This term means that a food, whether altered or not, contains 25 percent less of a nutrient or calories as compared to the reference food.
- Light – This descriptor can mean two things. A nutritionally altered product contains 1/3 fewer calories or 1/2 the fat of the reference food. If the food derives 50 percent or more of the calories from fat, the reduction must be 50 percent of the fat.
- More – A serving of food contains a nutrient that is at least 10 percent more of the Daily Value than the reference food.
- Percent Fat-Free – A product bearing this claim must be a low-fat or

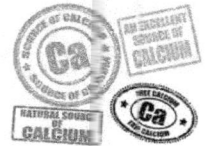

fat-free product. The claim must accurately represent the amount of fat present in 100 grams of the food. So, if the box of cookies you are picking up says 95 percent fat-free, it must contain 5 grams of fat per 100 grams.

ABOUT RESTAURANT TERMS:

TERMS THAT CAN BE NOT SO HEALTHY: what they really mean
- Scalloped: layered dish of vegetables and a sauce mixed with milk, butter and flour
- Au gratin: with cheese
- Buttered: added butter
- Basted: to moisten meat with fats or drippings
- Custard: eggs, cream, milk, butter and sugar used as a sweet sauce
- Fried: anything fried in oil
- Breaded: bread, eggs and butter combination
- Battered: fat, flour and water combination
- Creamy: added cream
- Crisp (savory): fried in butter or oil
- Tempura: batter coating of water, flour and eggs, fried
- Crisp (sweet): fried in butter and sugar
- Hollandaise: mixture of egg yolks and butter

TERMS THAT ARE USUALLY HEALTHY: what they really mean
- Au jus: in its own juice
- Sauté: cooking meat or vegetables in a very small amount of fat in a pan until brown
- Broiled: cooked under high heat
- Grilled: cooked over high heat to seal in natural juices
- Baked: over cooked, nothing added
- Braised: slow cooked in its own juice
- Lean: without added fat
- Roasted: cooking foods in radiant heat of oven or over open flame

- Poached: simmered in liquid
- Steamed: foods cooked over but not in boiling water

Other advice about eating out at restaurants:
- Ordering vegetarian options isn't always the healthiest option - vegetarian sandwiches and dishes are often laden with a hefty amount of mayo, oil, butter and other sauces that are loaded with extra fat and calories that completely negate the seemingly healthier option. Make sure the dish is prepared using any of the abovementioned healthy terms.
- Sandwiches are often loaded with mayo, bacon, cheese and other high calorie options. You are better off with just mustard, no cheese, fresh vegetables and a high quality protein source.
- Soups, like tomato and French onion, may not be the best option at some restaurants. Restaurants often add a ton of sodium and other fillers, like bread and cream, to make the soups more palatable and full of flavor. You are better off making your own soup at home, or ordering a salad. Speaking of salads....
- Some salads, like cobb and Caesar, tend to have more fat and calories than vegetables. Choose salads that consist of all vegetables and add some grilled chicken or salmon for some protein. Ask for dressing on the side to further reduce the calories.
- Turkey burger and turkey bacon aren't necessarily healthier than beef. Restaurants don't use as lean of a cut for the turkey burger so it is best to ask how lean the meat is for both beef and turkey (shoot for 90% or over). And turkey bacon is filled with sodium and artificial ingredients such as regular bacon, so it is best to look for bacon with no MSG or artificial ingredients.

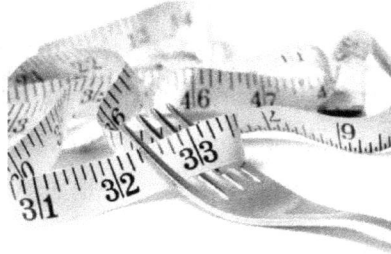

ABOUT DAILY CALORIC REQUIREMENT (DCR)

- One way to determine the number of calories your body requires each day is to ascertain your total caloric expenditure for the various activities you perform during the day and add to it the calories required for your basal metabolism.
- You could consult *My Fitness Pal,* which not only reports the calories contained in many foods, but also includes information about basal metabolism and the number of calories needed for many activities.

ABOUT BODY COMPOSITION:

- Knowing your percentage of body fat can help you to determine if your current nutrition and exercise program is helping you to lose fat and gain *lean body mass* in the correct proportions.
- The recommended average adult body fat is 15-18% for men and 22-25% for women.
- Using body weight and anthropometric measurements as indicators of changes in body fat is of unlimited value.
- You cannot determine if you are in good physical shape simply by stepping on a scale.
- The body mass index (BMI) is a poor predictor of percent body fat, fitness level or blood pressure.
- Hydrostatic weighing and BOD POD are the best options for assessing body fat.

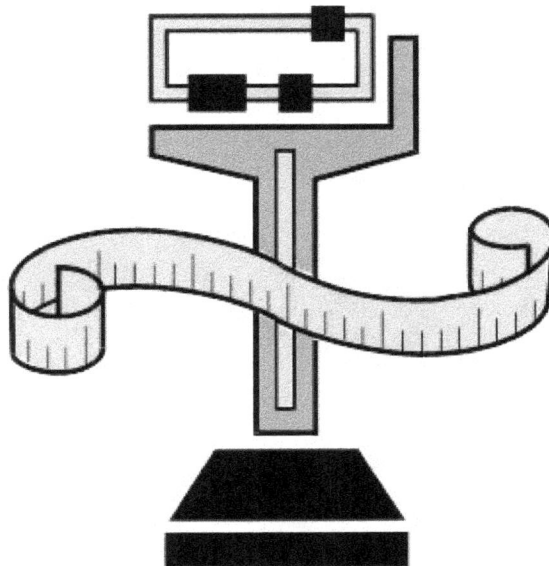

CHAPTER 4:
WHY!
(the philosophy governing the design of this plan)

When writing this book, our goal was to present you with a plethora of knowledge and a "How-To" guide. Additionally, we want you to understand why we eat the way we do, why we feel the way we do and why we want you to jump on board with us. Following something blindly, without knowledge of why, does not give you the freedom to have your own strength and peace. We aim to do just the opposite.

- A primary purpose, in addition to gaining weight, was to teach you how to eat properly. This involves choosing to eat the foods God put on earth and eliminating those you can purchase from a drive-through.
- Another primary objective was to teach you appropriate portion control so you will not overeat.
- There are no cheat days on this plan. If you're like most Americans, you have had your share of cheat days coming into this diet. We do recommend you try binging on "cheat foods" on day 22. Weigh yourself on the morning of day 22 and write down how you feel. Then let loose on day 22. Eat a lot. Eat a lot of junk. But then weigh yourself and write down how you felt on day 23. You'll like the comparisons.
- Research indicates it takes approximately 21 days to create a new habit. The plan is 21 days long to help you create a new way to eat.
- Because you are eating often, you will enjoy eating and feel satisfied.
- We want you to eat every three hours or so to keep your metabolism running high and burning lots of calories. Choosing quality proteins and fibrous vegetables forces your metabolism to run much higher than it would on the simple carbohydrates that man manufactures; hence more fat loss.
- Believe it or not, personal correspondence with Japan's top sumo wrestler revealed that they are only allowed to eat once a day so their metabolism with be as slow as possible.
- You are always ingesting protein, fat and carbohydrates so they are

always available for the body.

- You are always combining your carbohydrates with proteins to slightly lower the glycemic value of the carbohydrates and to provide a more stable blood sugar level in the body.
- Approximately 50-60% of the calories in this plan come from carbohydrates (good carbs) so you'll have plenty of energy.
- You will eat fruits earlier in the day for more energy but will switch to vegetables later in the day so as to not have excess sugar in the body during the resting state.
- The amount of protein needed daily is somewhere between 1 gram per kilogram of bodyweight and one pound of bodyweight for most, or about 20-30% of daily calories ingested.
- Each and every food contributes to bodily health so we are trying to vary the foods as much as possible to ensure maximum nutrient ingestion (taking into account buying and preparation convenience).
- We have tried to eliminate as many manufactured foods as possible (the stuff that has fattened our whole country).
- It has been theorized that separating the juice (sugary part) of the fruit from the pulp and fiber causes a huge glycemic spike so we are keeping our fruits in whole form.
- We have limited red meats to lower quantities to avoid excess hormones that are routinely injected into them, but have suggested more lean proteins such as bison and fish to provide lower hormone or even hormone-free quality proteins.
- Green tea is suggested because it provides energy from the caffeine, antioxidants for the immune system and metabolism boost.
- We ask that you consciously drink much more water than normal. The body is comprised of about 60% of water and it is critical to stay hydrated. For instance, in the time it takes to smile you create about 7

billion new cells in the liver alone. Every one of them needs water. Now you're convinced.

- Your body needs fat (in appropriate amounts) to provide you with energy and a feeling of fullness. Fats are also utilized in most of your daily bodily functions but should only comprise about 10-20% of the total calories.

- We have tried to eliminate trans fats, because they severely damage arteries and waistlines, by sticking to non-manufactured foods.

- This diet is also low on saturated fats, the ones that are killing people. They won't be killing you on this plan.

- This meal plan is not flawless. Some days we could have used another 2 grams of fiber, or a touch more of protein or fat, but that is by design. We are trying to create a good-tasting, pleasing, sound lifestyle change that promotes an optimal you. We are not trying to create a sterile meal plan or organic soybeans, tofu and celery stalks that come out to exactly 1200 calories. That was never our objective. We asked you to visualize the "after picture": the energetic, dynamic optimal you. Getting you there is our goal.

CHAPTER 5:

IT'S ON YOU

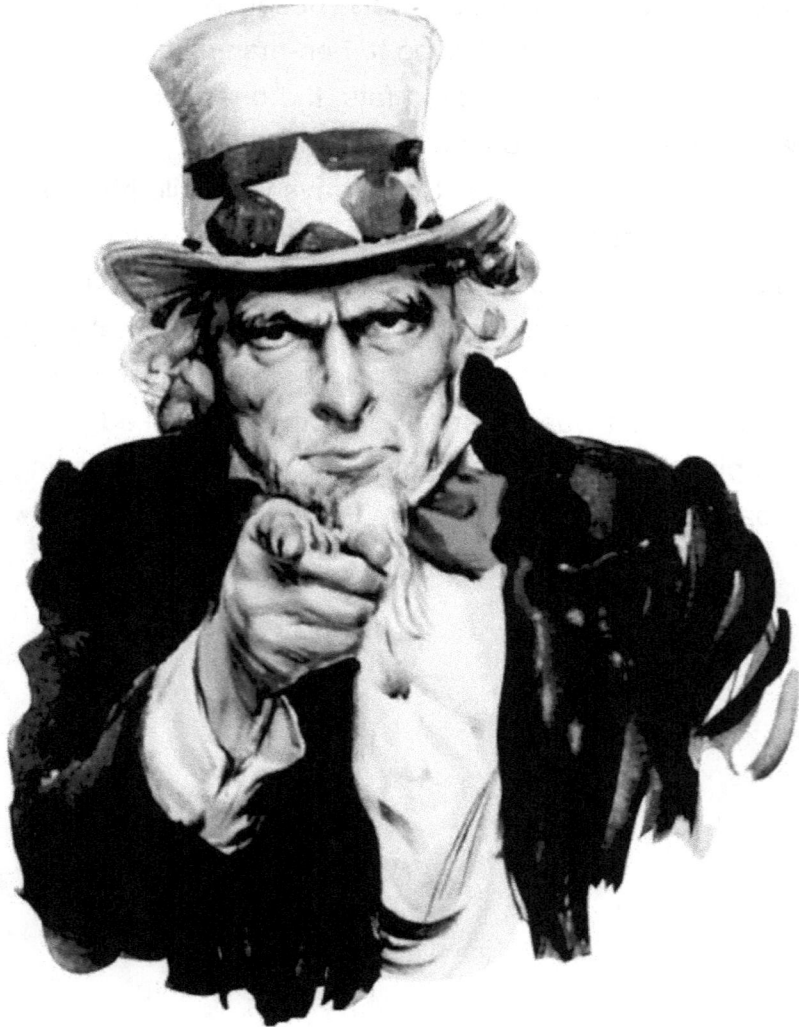

You now have 21 days of meticulously prepared meal plans. We've calculated the number of calories, the amount of protein, carbohydrates, fats, fiber, etc. for you. We have listed precise quantities and when to eat them. You have the knowledge of what proper nutrition is and how to plan further meal plans for yourselves. You also know that this plan has worked magic for others. It's quite the deal considering the price of this book—the pictures of us in our bigger days were worth more than that alone!

We're done. Now, it's your turn to see great things for yourself. Remember the words of Albert Einstein, "it's a preview of life's coming attractions."

Let nothing stop you in your quest.

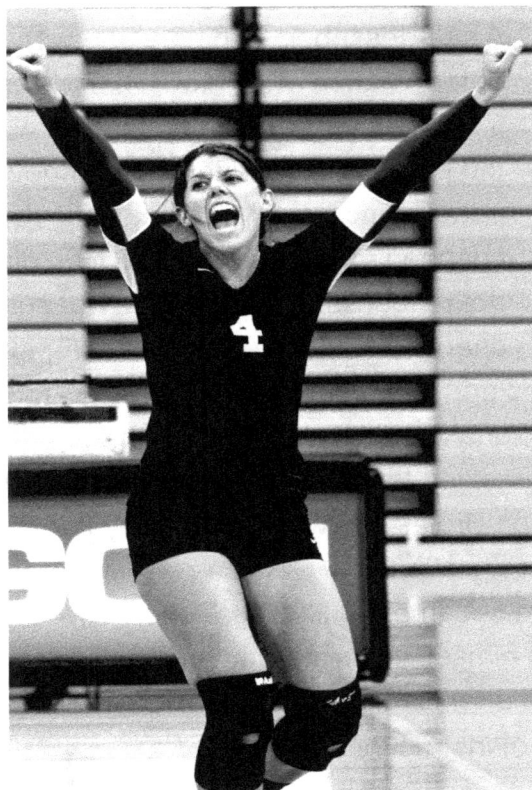

About the Authors

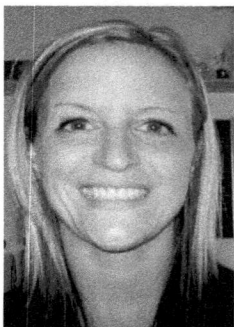

A graduate from Gonzaga University, **Liz Sambach**, B.S, C.S.C.S., A.C.E. P.T., is currently working on her Masters in Human Movement degree from the distinguished A.T. Still University. Having been fortunate to coach various sports teams at the junior college level and a range of high school athletes, Liz is also a licensed massage therapist and has worked with a variety of individuals from professional athletes to the average active adult. She currently holds a black belt in karate-do, is a multiple National Champion and is working towards a black belt in Judo.

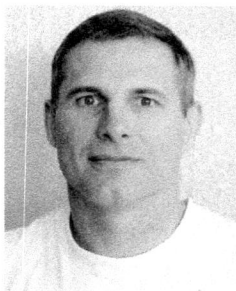

A self-described "ordinary guy with extraordinary determination" **Tim McClellan**, M.S., C.S.C.S., C.S.H. has distinguished himself worldwide during the past three decades as an innovator in the performance enhancement field. Among those he coached are more than 200 NFL players, 12 Olympic gold medalists, more than a dozen NCAA individual champions, 9 NCAA team champions, more than 200 NCAA All-Americans and National Champions of 17 different sports. Tim also coached at Arizona State University for 13 years and has worked with the USA Olympic wrestling team, the World Champion USA powerlifting team, and the Boston Bruins. He was honored by the National Strength and Conditioning Association in 1990 as a recipient of their President's Award. In 2012, Tim became certified as a sports hypnotist. A multiple National Champion himself in karate-do, Tim holds black belt ranks in five different martial arts. He has written numerous magazine articles and produced a variety of instructional videos.

For more information about the vitamins we mentioned:

- Vitamin A: http://lpi.oregonstate.edu/infocenter/vitamins/vitaminA/
- Vitamin D: http://lpi.oregonstate.edu/infocenter/vitamins/vitaminD/
- Vitamin E: http://lpi.oregonstate.edu/infocenter/vitamins/vitaminE/
- Vitamin K: http://lpi.oregonstate.edu/infocenter/vitamins/vitaminK/
- Thiamin: http://lpi.oregonstate.edu/infocenter/vitamins/thiamin/
- Riboflavin: http://lpi.oregonstate.edu/infocenter/vitamins/riboflavin/
- Niacin: http://lpi.oregonstate.edu/infocenter/vitamins/niacin/
- Vitamin B5:   http://lpi.oregonstate.edu/infocenter/vitamins/pa/
- Vitamin B6:   http://lpi.oregonstate.edu/infocenter/vitamins/vitaminB6/
- Vitamin B12:   http://lpi.oregonstate.edu/infocenter/vitamins/vitaminB12/
- Biotin: http://lpi.oregonstate.edu/infocenter/vitamins/biotin/
- Vitamin C: http://lpi.oregonstate.edu/infocenter/vitamins/vitaminC/
- Folic Acid: http://lpi.oregonstate.edu/infocenter/vitamins/fa/
- Boron: http://en.wikipedia.org/wiki/Boron
- Calcium: http://lpi.oregonstate.edu/infocenter/minerals/calcium/
- Chronium: http://lpi.oregonstate.edu/infocenter/minerals/chromium/
- Copper: http://lpi.oregonstate.edu/infocenter/minerals/copper/
- Iocine: http://lpi.oregonstate.edu/infocenter/minerals/iodine/
- Iron: http://lpi.oregonstate.edu/infocenter/minerals/iron/
- Magnesium: http://lpi.oregonstate.edu/infocenter/minerals/magnesium/
- Manganese: http://lpi.oregonstate.edu/infocenter/minerals/manganese/
- Mo ybdenum   http://lpi.oregonstate.edu/infocenter/minerals/molybdenum/
- Phosphate   http://en.wikipedia.org/wiki/Phosphate
- Potassium   http://lpi.oregonstate.edu/infocenter/minerals/potassium/
- Selenium   http://lpi.oregonstate.edu/infocenter/minerals/selenium/
- Zinc   http://lpi.oregonstate.edu/infocenter/minerals/zinc/

Also available from www.StrengthAndPeace.com

INNER STRENGTH INNER PEACE: Life-Changing Lessons From The World's Greatest, Volume 1

INNER STRENGTH INNER PEACE: Life-Changing Lessons From The World's Greatest, Volume 2

TRAINING PROGRAMS: Learn more about training programs similar to the ones the pros use

INSTRUCTIONAL DVDS

www.ingramcontent.com/pod-product-compliance
Lightning Source LLC
Chambersburg PA
CBHW080002280326
41935CB00013B/1721